CLINICAL SIMULATIONS: THE RIGHT WAY!
THE COMPLETE GUIDE FOR RESPIRATORY CARE PROVIDERS

BY C. J. PETERS, B.S., R.R.T.
Director of Student Services,
California College for Health Sciences
San Diego, California

SECOND PRINTING

CALIFORNIA COLLEGE FOR HEALTH SCIENCES
National City, CA 92050

CLINICAL SIMULATIONS: THE RIGHT WAY!
THE COMPLETE GUIDE FOR RESPIRATORY CARE PROVIDERS

BY C. J. PETERS, B.S., R.R.T.

Published By:

California College for Health Sciences
222 W. 24th Street
National City, CA 92050

First Printing 1990, Second Printing 1990

Library of Congress Cataloging-in-Publication Data
Peters, C.J., 1925-
Clinical Simulations - The Right Way! : The Complete Guide for Respiratory Care Providers / by C.J. Peters.
—1st ed.
p. cm.
Includes bibliographical references.
ISBN 0-931657-20-2
1. Respiratory therapy—Examinations, questions, etc. I. Title. (DNLM: 1. Respiratory Therapy — problems. WB P4812c)
RC735.I5P48 1990
616.2'0046—dc20
DNLM/DLC
for Library of Congress 90-1650 CIP

This book is dedicated to . . .

the thousands of working practitioners and students who make time for their families, careers, while furthering their professional educations.

TABLE OF CONTENTS

ABOUT THE AUTHOR

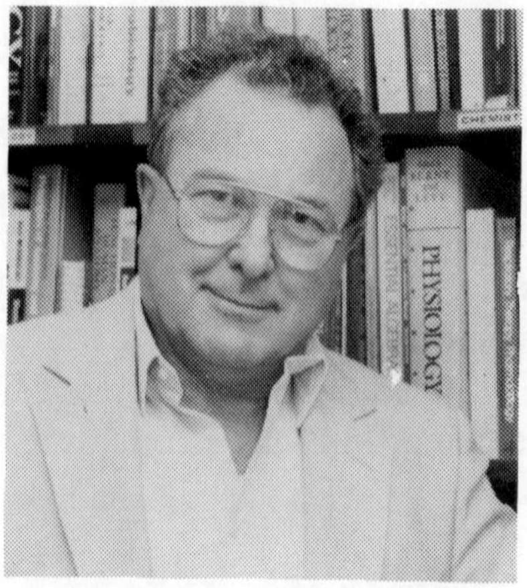

Charles J. Peters, B.S., RRT, is currently Director of Student Services at California College for Health Sciences (**CCHS**). He has lectured, coordinated, and helped thousands of students as a **CCHS** clinical instructor, clinical coordinator, and primary didactic lecturer since 1980.

Peters is a leading respiratory care instructor of students preparing for NBRC testing. He has lectured extensively across the United States to AARC affil-iates on examination preparation. He has also authored the **CCHS** NBRC Entry Level Preparation packet, the **CCHS** Written Registry Preparation packet, the **CCHS** Hyperbaric Oxygen Training Program, numerous **CCHS** educational units, and more.

Peters is a graduate of the University of Wisconsin and has been a respiratory therapist since 1972. He was one of the first professional, respiratory home-care providers in the 1970's.

ACKNOWLEDGEMENTS

My thanks for the encouragement and support of Dale Bean, RRT, Program Director and Kenneth Scheiderman, Chairman of the Board, both of California College for Health Sciences. I am particularly grateful to my very able colleague, Sandra Richey Wallace, Student Services Assistant Director at CCHS, who "fielded" a large part of my normal workload while this book was being written.

In addition, special recognition and thanks to Ms. Jaimi Warden whose sterling word processing skills and efforts were equal to the task of preparing the manuscript itself.

Charles J. Peters

Cover Design: Lorri Maida, Pacific Beach, CA.

INTRODUCTION

This book is written as a guide for the National Board for Respiratory Care (NBRC) candidate *as well as* an assessment tool for Program Directors, Respiratory Department Administrators and other Respiratory Care Providers.

It is a useful adjunct to the curriculum of respiratory care programs. Under the present essentials, you must have a reasonable portion of students be successful on the exam. Obviously, respiratory care programs have much more than "peripheral interest" in their graduates.

This text offers you a useful evaluation tool for progress of respiratory care students and for proficiency assessment of students and respiratory personnel directly involved in patient care.

For you the student, specifically preparing for the NBRC examinations, this book is vital to your success on the clinical simulations portion of the exam.

On that Saturday afternoon in June or December, having already worked through this presentation, there will be no surprises on the exam. In fact, you will be well prepared and confident.

We presume you are new to this...so we start at the absolute beginning. (And, if you're a seasoned respiratory care practitioner, it's a great refresher.)

Respiratory Clinical Simulation Testing: A Complete Guide

Introduction to Clinical Simulations

C.J. Peters, BS, RRT

INTRODUCTION TO THE CLINICAL SIMULATION FORMAT OF EXAMINATION

Vital to your success in this portion of the NBRC examination is proper preparation. These problems are designed to provide the tools to overcome this formidable obstacle. On that Saturday afternoon in June or December, you, by working through this presentation, will not be faced with any element of surprise. We assume you are a neophyte in this realm—hence we start at the absolute beginning.

Basic Premises

1. You may order, suggest, recommend or change whatever you like in the management of the patient. You are to assume there is a physician available who will request your assistance and will sign any orders, if so needed. This is not the case, probably, in your actual practice of respiratory care, but, for these exercises and on examination day, you may do what you wish. YOU are in command!

2. Management of the patient must conform to clinical reality. Many of the distractors (wrong answers) offered would be impossible to perform, logistically impossible, clinically unreal, and too time consuming to be of value. These factors must be considered as you work through this exercise.
Criteria to apply to suspicious distractors:

a. Can it be done in the patient's present situation?
b. Are the necessary tubes, catheters, instrumentation etc. at hand to accomplish the test/procedure?
c. Would test results be available immediately to be of benefit in the face of a potentially life threatening situation?
d. Could the patient perform an effort dependent test?
e. Would the test/procedure require moving a critically ill patient?
f. Is the test/procedure in the mainstream of respiratory care? (i.e., does it appear on the outline of the written registry exam?)

We have provided a glossary of terms to familiarize you with those commonly used distractors and terms which are obtuse in nature. (Appendix A)

3. Management of clinical problems must follow the accepted criteria found in the body of respiratory care literature. It also must follow the generally accepted, conservative approach to patient management. This may, or may not, be the case in your hospital, but for this exercise and examination day — follow this premise!

4. A misstep with a latent image marker pen is irretrievable! Follow instructions carefully and cautiously. Your route through the exam is not in alphabetical or numerical order. A factor to reckon with is paging forward and backward as you traverse the problem and still stay on course.

5. Progress through an exam is not by page number or alphabetical order. You will be moving forward and backward as the directions send you. Be prepared to do much "thumbing" back and forth. A correctly traversed problem will have several blank sections. You have not overlooked sections of the exam. These are alternate routes you were successful in evading. Again, follow the directions exactly!

THE MECHANICS OF CLINICAL SIMULATION PROBLEMS

Each problem begins with a scenario. Here, you are placed in the clinical situation and given a general sketch of the patient. It, invariably begins with, "You are a respiratory therapist in..."

Sample Scenario

You are a p.m. shift respiratory therapist in a 300-bed community hospital. Charles Wills, the 30 year old driver of a car involved in a multi-car accident, is brought to the emergency room. You are paged by the emergency room nurse, who says the on-call physician is on the way to the hospital and requests you to assist in the management of the patient. After entering the emergency room you determine the patient is confused, approximatley 184 cm (6 ft) tall and weighs 175 lbs. (79.5 kg).
The scenario is preceded by the following declarative: **"NOW GO TO SECTION A".**

From here-on-out your track will no longer be in alphabetical order.

An information gathering section will have as the last response:
"When you have completed your selections in this section, develop A-21, B-13, J-16 etc.".

Using the latent image developing pen, develop the example below:

<u>Example</u>

Decision making sections will direct you as you uncover your selection.

<u>Example</u>

B-3 Set the FIO_2 at 0.8

(develop with your pen)

Note the double asterisk. This indicates the end of the statement. Be sure you see the double asterisk before moving on. It is possible to miss key information by making this simple, mechanical error.

Information gathering sections allow you to: **"Select as many as you feel are indicated in this section."**

Decision making sections require you to, [**Choose only one, unless you are directed to "make another selection in this section".**]
If you err, you must choose again, at the cost of points—depending on the severity of the error.

MAP AND ROUTES THROUGH THE EXAM

Below is a typical map of a clinical simulation problem. The optimal route is a direct, vertical straight line descent through the problem. This route rewards the candidate with the highest score. The alternate routes through the map will yield less points. The construction of the problem is such that alternate routes always lead back to the main route.

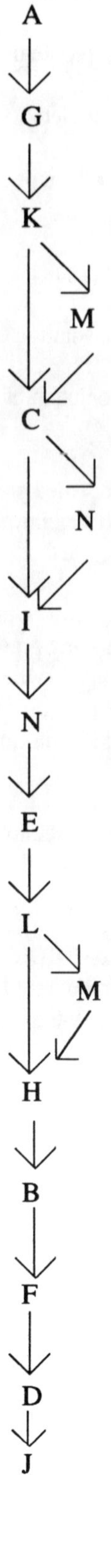

SCORING CRITERIA

Each choice you make is weighted according to the criteria listed below:

+ 3 Of central importance toward resolution of the patient's immediate problem

+ 2 Strongly facilitative towards resolution of the problem

+ 1 Mildly facilitative towards resolution of the problem

0 Neither helpful or harmful in the care of the patient, or could be of help only in remote, secondary situations

- 1 Mildly harmful towards the resolution of the problem

- 2 Seriously harmful or detrimental towards the solution of the problem

- 3 Gravely harmful or detrimental towards the solution of the problem, possibly contraindicated

In the answers and explanations portion located in the sealed portion of each problem you will score each section and arrive at a total score. The clinical simulation examinations are not numerically graded, except for achievement of a minimum passing score. Any score above that is a pass—anything below that figure is a fail.

There are minimum passing level (MPL) scores which must be achieved on both decision making and information gathering sections on the actual NBRC exams. A passing grade is attained by correctly responding at a rate of approximately 70%. Fortunately, the scoring is cumlative on the complete set of ten problems. This allows you to regain points lost on a problem where you have had difficulties. If you achieve the minimum pass level on the cumulative total for each category of response (decision making simulation portion of the NBRC credentialing examinations.

The distinction between information gathering and decision making has been eliminated on our process problems. This was done to simplify the scoring process and allow you to quickly and easily assess your skill as you proceed through the sample examinations.

If you inadvertently begin to uncover a response on the NBRC exams, and then decide against it, don't leave it partially uncovered. The NBRC grading format is programmed to disallow all positive scoring beyond that point in all remaining sections of that problem. The computer interprets this as "peeking" and punishes you accordingly. Uncover the answer in its entirety and take the consequences. In this manner, you stand a chance of making up the lost points in the overall scoring. Leaving a partially uncovered answer carries the risk of losing a greater number of points which makes recovery that much more difficult.

Below is a sample of an information gathering section and its scoring. This section is from a problem occurring on a Myesthenia Gravis patient who is being mechanically ventilated. (use your latent image pen to develop)

SECTION H

Twenty-four hours later you are standing at the bedside of Mrs. Smith and note the high pressure alarm sounding with each breath. To determine the cause of the problem, which of the following would you evaluate?

Select as many as you feel are indicated in this section.	**scoring**	**comment**
H-1 Arterial blood gases		(H-1) of no help
H-2 Chest auscultation		(H-2) evidence of pneumothorax
H-3 Negative inspiratory force		(H-3) a weaning parameter
H-4 Vital capacity		(H-4) self explanatory
H-5 Pulse and blood		(H-5) condition is deteriorating
H-6 Resistance to negative ventilation		(H-6) eliminates a ventilatory problem
H-7 Deep tendon reflexes		(H-7) of no help
H-8 Ventilator settings		(H-8) a possible cause
H-9 Peripheral muscle strength		(H-9) the patient is paralyzed
H-10 Lactate levels		(H-10) of no help
H-11 Diagnostic chest percussion		(H-11) indirect evidence of pneumothorax
H-12 Capability of passing a suction catheter		(H-12) eliminates ET tube obstruction
H-13 Peak expiratory flow		(H-13) self explanatory
H-14 Complete blood cell count (CBC)		(H-14) of no help
H-15 Oxygen consumption (Vo_2)		(H-15) time consuming and of no help
H-16 Functional residual capacity		(H-16) self explanatory
H-17 Position of trachea		(H-17) evidence of pneumothorax

Below is a typical decision making section involving the myesthenia patient as above. The proper decision is to intubate and ventilate, as indicated for a Myesthenia Gravis patient with a tidal volume of 175 ml. With this blood gas data, the patient is in impending ventilatory failure.

SECTION J

Mrs. Smith's vital capacity is 0.8L (25% of predicted), tidal volume 175 ml. respiratory rate 34/min. pulse 120/min., BP 140/110 mmHg, stat arterial blood gas results reveal FIO_2 0.40. PO_2 58, pH 7.36, HCO_3^- 25, and PCO_2 46. Which of the following would you now recommend?

Choose only one, unless you are directed to "make another selection in this section"	**scoring**	**comments**
J-1 Intubation and administration of CPAP at 5cmH_2O, FIO_2 0.5		(J-1) potentially dangerous to an apneic patient
J-2 Increasing the FIO_2 to 1.0		(J-2) not harmful, but not helpful. Direction is to an alternate route.
J-3 Maintaining present level of therapy and continuing to monitor		(J-3) some positive action required.
J-4 Intubation and mechanical ventilation		(J-4) "impending" ventilatory failure is the indicator.
J-5 Increasing FIO_2 to 0.5		(J-5) potentially harmful.

THE SCOPE OF THE EXAM

The NBRC clinical simulation examination will be ten problems from the list below. The first seven are the "core". The remaining four are a mixed bag. The design of the problems in this packet is such to provide a valid preparatory base. There are 11 problems covering a selection from each category of the "core" and samples from 8, 9, and 10.

1.	COPD	-pre/post operative -mechanical ventilation	-rehabilitation
2.	COPD	-home care	-PFT evaluation
3.	Trauma		
4.	Cardiovascular		
5.	Neurologic		
6.	Pediatric		
7.	Neonate/infant		
8.	Misc.	-hypothermia -drug overdose	
9.	Misc.	-burn -CO poisoning	-Pickwickian
10.	Misc.	-surgical	-etc.

RECOMMENDED READING

Recommended reading is as follows:
Burton and Hodgkin:Respiratory Care. A Guide to Clinical Practice. 2nd edition. J.B. Lipincott 1985 Philadelphia. Chapters 28-33 and appendix D.

Shapiro:Clinical Application of Respiratory Care. Third edition. Year Book Medical Publishers, Chicago 1985. Chapters 28-33.

Mitchel: Synopsis of Pulmonary Disease. Third edition 1982.
C.V. Mosby. St. Louis.

INSTRUCTIONS FOR THE USE OF THIS PREPARATION PACKET!

Here is how we would like you to proceed.

1. Familiarize yourself with the glossary of commonly used terminology of clinical simulation problems . Most of them are distractors, some could be terms you might be unfamiliar with at first glance.

2. Work through the first exam under simulated test conditions. Don't unseal the answers and explanations section until you have finished.

3. Upon completion, open the answer and explanations portion. This section is arranged in optimal route order. Score each section as you go. Alternate route sections are at the back of the booklet. The final page has a recap of the scoring and the map through the problem.

4. Return to the exam, itself, and uncover all answers. In this manner, you will get a feel for the flow of the exam and, to review your thought process on any distractors you selected.

Our wish for you is, "Success on the NBRC exam". Luck is helpful, but preparation and luck go hand in hand. We think you will see steady improvement in your scores as you work through the individual problems. So, "Good Luck" after good preparation—and be a succesful registered respiratory therapist.

C.J. Peters
CCHS 1989

GLOSSARY OF TERMS AND COMMONLY USED DISTRACTORS APPLICABLE TO CLINICAL SIMULATION EXAMINATIONS

anaerobic metabolism	a treadmill test term denoting exercise level where metabolic acidosis first appears.
angiograms	always a distractor
antibody titer	requires days to complete
appearance of skin	an indicator of perfusion/cardiac-output/shock, fever, etc.
atropine	the indicated drug for the treatment of bradycardia and as a bronchodilator, where others have caused an adverse reation
Babinski Reflex	always a distractor; it is a neurologic indicator. It is very painful to a conscious patient.
basal metabolic rate	a measure of oxygen uptake; useful only in advanced exercise studies
blood culture	always a distractor; it is an indicator of blood infection when positive.
bowel sounds	always a distractor; of no value for respiratory assessment or treatment.
brain scan (CAT, angio, magnetic)	always a distractor; of no value for respiratory assessment or treatment
bronchogram	a radiopaque lung scan to determine bronchiectasis; usually a distractor
capillary refill (color of nailbeds)	an indicator of adequate perfusion/cardiac output (nail bed is compressed—watch for reperfusion)
carboxyhemoglobin	of value only in the assessment of carbon monoxide poisoning
cardiac enzymes	of value only if myocardial infection is suspected; usually a distractor
carotid massage	massaging the carotid arteries, below the ear to speed up bradycardia.
cerebrospinal fluid pressure	always a distractor
clotting time (prothrombin)	always a distractor; of no value to respiratory assessment or treatment
corneal reflex (pupillary response)	an indicator of oxygenation of the lower brainstem, usually a distractor

colloid osmotic pressure	usually a distractor; an indicator of pulmonary edema of pulmonic origin
culture and sensitivity (sputum)	requires 12 hours for final results
deep tendon reflex (response to pain)	always a distractor; of no value to respiratory assessment or treatment
dextrose stick	usually a distractor; of no value to respiratory assessment or treatment
dynamic compliance	usually a distractor; a choice only in computation of compliance
electroencephalogram (EEG)	always a distractor
fluid challenge	usually a distractor; only applicable to determine hypovolemia in conjunction with Swan-Ganz data
G.I. (series, scan)	always a distractor
gag reflex	always a distractor
genitalia	always a distractor
graded exercises	only applicable to rehabilitation procedures
heart sounds	always a distractor
Herring-Breur reflex	always a distractor
inotropic drugs	applicable only to improve cardiac output; usually a distractor(also, chronotropic drugs,dromotrophic drugs)
intracranial pressure	a choice only when head injury; patient is mechanically ventilated
intraocular pressure	always a distractor
lactate level	only applicable to determine anaerobic metabolism; usually a distractor
lateral neck X-Ray	only applicable to diagnosis of epiglottitis and croup
lidocaine	applicable to treatment of premature ventricular contractions
long bone fracture	only applicable to pulmonary fat emboli
lung scan (ventilation/perfusion xenon, radiopaque, etc.)	only applicable to differentiate pulmonary emboli from V/Q mismatch; requires moving the patient

moro reflex	always a distractor, except in neonatology; arms cross chest when startled
Mueller-Hinton test	always a distractor; it is a test for antibiotic sensitivity and n. gonorrhea.
myelogram	always a distractor
P-50	usually a distractor; only a choice where O_2 carrying capability is a factor
pedal edema	an indicator of right heart failure secondary to chronic pulmonary disease
PPD (positive protein derivative)	always a distractor; only applicable as test for tuberculosis
range of motion (ROM)	usually a distractor; only applicable to pulmonary rehabilitation context
serum electrolytes	only of value where potassium is being infused or intensive care situation where abnormal K^+ results are a possibility
spinal tap	always a distractor
swallow, ability to	only of value in neurological disease; i.e. M. Gravis, or Guillaine-Barre, etc.
tine test	always a distractor; a test for tuberculosis
toxin screen	always a distractor; a battery of tests for poisons; requires weeks
urine, urinalysis (sodium, output, culture)	always a distractor
Weil-Felix test	a test for Proteus and Ricksetsia; usually a distractor

Mike Kowalski

Clinical Simulation #1

Problem

MIKE KOWALSKI

You are a staff respiratory therapist in a 320-bed protestant religion sponsored community hospital. At the start of the day shift you are paged by the hospital's pulmonary service. They request you see a newly admitted patient. The only information you are given is that the patient is in respiratory distress.

NOW GO TO SECTION A

SECTION A

On the pulmonary floor you meet Mike Kowalski. He is a 56 year old male, somewhat overweight, ruddy complexion, and is sitting on the side of his bed. He is in a state of panic. His principal statement is, "can't breathe!" Your initial evaluation of this patient would include which of the following physical findings?

Choose as many as you feel are indicated in this section.

A-1	Pulse	98/min.**
A-2	Ability to swallow	
A-3	Skin assessment	Florid, diaphoretic, slightly dusky**
A-4	Chest auscultation	Rales, rhonchi, in lower and middle lobes**
A-5	Deep tendon reflexes	
A-6	Chest configuration	Hyperinflated "barrel" shaped**
A-7	Pupillary reaction	
A-8	Bowel sounds	
A-9	Medications taken at home	Theo-Dur capsules QID**
A-10	Gag reflex	

A-11 Posture	[illegible]
A-12 Sensorium	[illegible]
A-13 Capillary refill	Normal**
A-14 Respiratory rate and pattern	24/min. Shallow, using accessory muscles**
A-15 Hering-Breur reflex	
A-16 Allen test	
A-17 Color of lips and mucosa	Slight cyanosis**
A-18 Heart sounds	
A-19 Diagnostic chest percussion	Resonant**
A-20 Temperature	39 C**
When you have **completed** your selections, **then develop A-21**	Go to Section D**

SECTION B

The attending physician asks for your recommendations on a more complete evaluation of Mr. Kowalski's pulmonary situation. Which would you suggest?

Choose as many as you feel are indicated in this section.

B-1	Blood urine nitrogen (BUN)	
B-2	Electroencephalogram	
B-3	Electrocardiogram	Sinus tachycardia rate 110/min.**
B-4	Complete blood count (CBC) and differential	Hb 16.5 gm%, WBC 18,000cu. mm, RBC 5.8cu mm elevated neutrophil count**
B-5	Blood culture	
B-6	Arterial blood gases	Obtained stat pH 7.33, PCO_2 59 mmHg, mmHg, HCO_3^- 32 mEq/l, % sat. 91, FIO_2 0.28**
B-7	Serum electrolytes	K^+ 3 meQ/l, NA^+ 136 mEq/l, CL 96 mEq/l, HCO_3^- 32 mEq/l**
B-8	Serum albumin	
B-9	Chest x-rays	Depressed diaphragms, increased vascular markings. Bilateral densities lower lobes, lingula and middle lobes.**
B-10	Cardiac enzymes	
B-11	% Saturation carboxyhemogloblin	
B-12	Urine culture	

B-13 Ventilation/perfusion scan

B-14 Sputum cultures for gram stain and sensitivity

B-15 Lactic acid level

B-16 Negative inspiratory force

B-17 Sputum specimen for cytology

B-19 **When you have completed your** selections in this section, then develop B-19

SECTION C

Initial blood gas values, prior to oxygen administration are pH 7.33, PCO_2 61 mmHg, PO_2 59 mmHg, HCO_3^- 32 mEq/l, % saturation 87%.

Of the following, which would you recommend to deliver oxygen therapy?

Choose only one, unless you are directed to "make another selection in this section."

C-1 Nasal Cannula 2 L/min.

C-2 Oxygen mask 5 L/min.

C-3 40% Venturi mask

C-4 28% Venturi mask

C-5 Partial rebreather mask, flow sufficient to keep reservoir bag from collapsing

SECTION D

Which would be your first suggestion upon arrival of the attending physician?

Choose only one, unless you are directed to "make another selection in this section."

D-1 Admit to the intensive care unit immediately

D-2 Obtain arterial blood gases

D-3 Administer acetylcysteine followed by chest physical therapy

D-4 Administer aerosolized albuterol followed by ultrasonic aerosol therapy

D-5 Obtain sputum for laboratory assessment

SECTION E

Twenty minutes later, Mr. Kowalski is alert and oriented. The physician requests you obtain a pulmonary history and report back to him.

Which would you include in your findings?

Choose as many as you feel are indicated in this section.

E-1 Cough?

E-2 Occupation?

E-3 Sputum production?

E-4 History of pulmonary infections?

E-5 Family history of cardio-pulmonary disease?

E-6 Family history of asthma?

E-7 Sleeping posture?

E-8 Parents' cause of death?

E-9 Daily activities?

E-10 Smoking history?

E-11 Other members of immediate family who smoke?

E-12 Social activities?

E-13 Number of children?

E-14 Allergies to drugs?

E-15 Night "sweats"?

E-16 Swelling of feet and ankles?

E-17 Family history of digestive disease?

E-18 Alcohol consumption?

E-19 **When you have completed your selections in this section, then develop E-19**

SECTION F

Twenty minutes later, Mr. Kowalski's blood pressure is 180/110 mmHg. ABG's are pH 7.29, PCO_2 68 mmHg, PO_2 68 mmHg, % saturation 84%, HCO_3^-32 mEq/l. The attending physician asks for your recommendation.

Which would you choose?

Choose only one, unless you are directed to "make another selection in this section."

F-1 Administer O_2 via 28% venturi mask

F-2 Discontinue oxygen therapy

F-3 Administer O_2 nasal cannula at 2 L/min.

F-4 Administer O_2 via non-rebreather mask

F-5 Intubate, adminster 40% O_2 via large volume heated nebulizer

SECTION G

The physician orders appropriate antibiotic and other therapies to treat the patient. He asks for your recommendation on any further respiratory therapy that would benefit the patient.

Which would you recommend?

Choose only one, unless you are directed to "make another selection in this section."

G-1 Incentive spirometry with breathing retaining

G-2 Increase FIO_2 to 0.40 via venturi mask

G-3 Bronchodilator therapy followed by postural drainage, percussion and vibration

Physician agrees, go to Section K**

G-4 IPPB Q4 hours with aerosolized solumedrol

G-5 No therapy is indicated

SECTION H

Three days later, the attending physician deems Mike's progress sufficient to warrant discharge from the hospital. The physician asks your suggestions as to Mike's care after leaving the hospital.

Which would you recommend?

Choose only one, unless you are directed to "make another selection in this section."

H-1 Order home oxygen therapy 1 L/min. via transtracheal route

H-2 Refer to the hospital's pulmonary rehabilitation program

H-3 Refer to the county visiting nurse service for ongoing care

H-4 Schedule patient for physician's office visits once per month

H-5 Schedule patient for pulmonary outpatient clinic visits once per month

SECTION J

Based on the results of the pulmonary workup and previous assessments, what would be your report on Mr. Kowalski's pulmonary disease?

Choose only one, unless you are directed to "make another selection in this section."

J-1 Mild obstructive disease, predominant bronchitic involvement, responsive to bronchodilator

J-2 Moderate obstructive disease, predominant emphysema involvement, non-responsive to bronchodilator

J-3 Moderate obstructive disease, predominant bronchitic involvement, responsive to bronchodilator

J-4 Severe obstructive disease, mixed emphysema/bronchitis involvement, non-responsive to bronchodilator

Physician agrees, go to Section H**

J-5 Severe obstructive disease, predominant asthmatic involvement, non-responsive to bronchodilator

SECTION K

Mr. Kowalski responds favorably to therapy. Three days later, the attending physician requests pulmonary function tests to classify Mike's pulmonary disease and its degree of progression.

Which tests would you recommend?

Choose as many as you feel are indicated in this section.

K-1 P-50	Not determined**
K-2 Arterial blood gases	pH 7.38, PCO_2 52 mmHg, PO_2 56 mmHg, HCO_3^- 29, % O_2 sat. 91%, FIO_2 0.21**
K-3 Plethysmography	TLC 5.9 liters (112% of predicted)**
K-4 Pulmonary stress test	Ordered**
K-5 Oxygen uptake	Not determined**
K-6 Diffusion of the lung carbon monoxide (D_LCO)	18 ml/min/mmHg (74% of predicted)**
K-7 Closing volumes	[illegible]
K-8 FEV_1/FVC %	46%**

K-9	Nitrogen balance study	
K-10	FEV_1, pre- and post-bronchodilator	Before—1.23 L, After — 1.27 **
K-11	Bronchogram	
K-12	**When you have completed your selections in this section, then develop K-12**	Go to Section J**

Mike Kowalski

Clinical Simulation #1

Answers, Explanations, and Scoring

MIKE KOWALSKI

This problem involves you in the care of a COPD patient, initially, in an acute situation. You are required to make decisions to relieve his immediate symptoms, evaluate his pulmonary status, and recommend tests which would be of value in his course of treatment. Finally, you must test and classify his COPD and participate in post-discharge planning.

SECTION A

Positive Scoring:

A-1, A-12, A-14, and A-17 Are all indicators that our patient is in a state of hypoxemia/hypoxia—probably severe.

A-3, A-4, and A-20 Are indicators that our patient has underlying infection.

A-6, A-9, A-11, and A-19, Are all indicators that our patient has underlying COPD.

A-13 Is an indicator there is peripheral perfusion, hence, adequate cardiac output.

The positive scoring depicts a COPD patient in throes of an acute pulmonary infection. The choices are those that encompass a reasonably thorough evaluation without resorting to empirical data or equipment other than your eyes, hands, and stethoscope.

Zero Scoring:

A-16 An Allen test, is of no immediate use. It might be in the near future—hence, the zero score.

Negative Scoring:

A-2, A-5, A-7, A-8, and A-15 are neurologic tests. There is no information implying neurological deficit.

A-10 and A-18 Are outside the scope of a pulmonary assessment.

All negative choices would be redundant and time wasting. In some cases, they would inflict pain.

	Possible	My Score
A-1	+ 1	+1
A-2	- 1	
A-3	+ 2	+2
A-4	+ 2	+2
A-5	- 2	
A-6	+ 1	+1
A-7	- 1	
A-8	- 1	
A-9	+ 1	+1
A-10	- 2	
A-11	+ 1	+1
A-12	+ 2	+2
A-13	+ 1	+1
A-14	+ 2	+2
A-15	- 2	
A-16	0	
A-17	+ 1	+1
A-18	- 1	
A-19	+ 2	+2
A-20	+ 1	+1
Total	**16**	17

SECTION D

Positive Scoring:

D-2 Is the preferable "first" choice. This would provide a baseline indicator of the patient's ability to ventilate on his own. It will also be an indicator of the progression and compensation of his pulmonary impairment.

Zero Scoring:

Choices D-3, D-4, and D-5 Would all be contributory to, and of benefit to the patient, although not the "first" action, to be taken. You are not penalized for this reason.

Negative Scoring:

D-1 This would be premature. The administration of oxygen could, possibly prevent such a drastic measure.

	Possible	My Score
D-1	- 3	
D-2	+ 3	+ 3
D-3	0	
D-4	0	0
D-5	0	
Total	+ 3	+ 3

SECTION C

Positive Scoring:

The blood gas data depicts acute ventilatory failure superimposed on chronic ventilatory failure.

C-1 and C-4 Are safe dosages to initiate oxygen therapy without risking oxygen induced hypoventilation. Oxygen induced hypoventilation would pose a risk with a patient assuredly a long term CO_2 retainer.

Negative Scoring:

C-2, C-3, and C-5 Are unsafe dosages and could cause grave harm to the patient (oxygen induced ventilation).

	Possible	My Score
C-1	+ 3	+3
C-2	- 2	
C-3	- 1	
C-4	+ 3	
C-5	- 3	
Total	**+ 3**	+3

SECTION F

Positive Scoring:

The patient has deteriorated as a result of excessive dosage of oxygen in the preceding Section C.

F-1 and F-3 Will reverse this adverse reaction.

Negative Scoring:

F-2 Would cause the patient great harm. He needs oxygen—but not quite as much.

F-4 Is more of the same—too much oxygen.

F-5 Intubation indications are not present. Also, 40% oxygen is excessive—as above.

	Possible	My Score
F-1	+ 2	
F-2	- 3	
F-3	+ 2	
F-4	- 3	
F-5	- 3	
Total	+ 3	

SECTION B

Positive Scoring:

B-4 A CBC would provide baseline information as to adequacy of the O_2 transport mechanism and clues to the patient's infection.

B-6, B-9, and B-14 Are central to the patient's treatment.

B-17 and B-18 Are rule-out measures as lung cancer or tuberculosis as possible, underlying factors.

Zero Scoring:

B-7 Serum electrolytes neither contribute nor detract from the patient's course of treatment.

Negative Scoring:

B-1, B-2, B-3, B-5, B-8, B-10, and B-12 All are outside the scope of a pulmonary workup.

B-11 There is no evidence of carbon monoxide poisoning.

B-13 A V/Q scan is redundant as there is no evidence that lung perfusion might be contributing to the problem.

B-15 Redundant! The blood gases document this is not a contributory factor.

B-16 Is a weaning procedure.

	Possible	My Score
B-1	- 2	
B-2	- 2	
B-3	- 3	-3
B-4	+ 1	+1
B-5	- 1	
B-6	+ 2	+2
B-7	0	0
B-8	- 2	
B-9	+ 3	+3
B-10	- 2	
B-11	- 2	
B-12	- 2	
B-13	- 2	
B-14	+ 2	+2
B-15	- 2	
B-16	- 1	
B-17	+ 1	
B-18	+ 1	
Total	**10**	5

SECTION E

Positive Scoring:

E-1, E-3, E-9, E-10, E-15, and E-16 Are factors occurring as a direct result and confirm a definite COPD profile.

E-2, E-4, E-7, E-8, and E-18 Are background factors that contributed to the patient's profile of COPD.

E-5, E-6, E-8, and E-14 Are hereditary factors which should be covered in any examination. They may or may not provide clues.

E-11 Is a factor—living with a smoker has been definitely linked to COPD.

Zero Scoring:

E-12 and E-13 Only under very remote circumstances would these contribute to a pulmonary history.

Negative Scoring:

Only E-17 would be beyond the realm of a pulmonary history.

	Possible	My Score
E-1	+2	+2
E-2	+1	+1
E-3	+2	+2
E-4	+1	+1
E-5	+1	+1
E-6	+1	+1
E-7	+1	+1
E-8	+1	+1
E-9	+2	+2
E-10	+2	+2
E-11	+1	+1
E-12	0	
E-13	0	—
E-14	+1	+1
E-15	+2	+2
E-16	+2	+2
E-17	- 1	—
E-18	+1	+1
Total	**21**	21

SECTION G

Positive Scoring:

G-3 The indications for postural drainage, percussion and vibration are present. Bronchodilator therapy would be a useful adjunct.

G-4 IPPB would be useful and is indicated for mobilization of secretions. Solumedrol (a corticosteroid) is not indicated, but would not harm the patient—hence the lower scoring value.

Negative Scoring:

G-1 Is only indicated for postoperative prophylaxis of atelectasis.

G-2 Oxygenation is presently within satisfactory limits (Section B-6) and we already know the patient is subject to oxygen induced hypoventilation.

G-5 Failure to address the problem of pooled, retained secretions in a pulmonary sepsis situation could cause the patient grave harm.

	Possible	My Score
G-1	- 3	
G-2	- 3	
G-3	+ 3	+3
G-4	+ 1	
G-5	- 3	
Total	**+ 3**	+3

SECTION K

Positive Scoring:

K-2 Arterial blood gases are necessary not only for a resting baseline, but are determinants of such items as payment for home oxygen, disabilities, etc.

K-3 Documents accurately the degree of hyperinflation. 112% of predicted quantifies hyperinflation as moderate to severe.

K-4 A pulmonary stress test will document the extent of Mike's pulmonary reserves, and possibilities of extending his activities after discharge.

K-6 Is critical to determine the differential between the emphysema/bronchitis involvement of his COPD—25 mL/min./Hg is normal.

K-8 Is the classic assessment of the presence of and degree of progression of obstructive disease.

K-10 Will assign a degree of reversibility of the pulmonary disease and guide bronchodilator therapy.

Negative Scoring:

K-1 Would not yield data helpful to classify, nor to what degree the disease had progressed.

K-5 Also of no help.

K-7 Concerns air trapping—of little value to obtain the stated goals.

K-9 Is a metabolic study.

K-11 Is a study to determine bronchiectasis, for which there is no evidence.

	Possible	My Score
K-1	- 2	
K-2	+ 2	+2
K-3	+ 1	+1
K-4	+ 2	+2
K-5	- 2	
K-6	+ 2	
K-7	- 1	
K-8	+ 2	+2
K-9	- 2	
K-10	+ 2	+2
K-11	- 1	
Total	11	9

SECTION J

Positive Scoring:

J-4 Is correct as follows:

1. FEV_1/FVC % is drastically reduced.
2. Blood gas analysis reveals sharply depressed P_aO_2, abnormally high PCO_2, and significant metabolic compensation.
4. Hyperinflation is significantly present (TLC 112% predicted).
5. The D_LCO is reduced significantly to denote destruction of lung tissue and vascularity (emphysema) as well as bronchitis (production of 1 1/2 cups of sputum per day).
6. There was very little response to bronchodilator indicating the absence of an asthmatic component.

	Possible	My Score
J-1	- 3	
J-2	- 3	
J-3	- 3	
J-4	+ 3	+3
J-5	- 3	
Total	**+ 3**	+ 3

SECTION H

Positive Scoring:

H-2 Although Mike's disease is severe, there are options, procedures, modalities which can enhance his quality of life. These should be made available to him.

After his disease has stabilized, a rehab program is positioned much better to make decisions as to his future.

Negative Scoring:

H-1 Mike would not qualify for payment by third parties for home oxygen therapy with the available blood gas data.

H-3 Visiting nurse services, usually, do not include respiratory services that Mike would need.

H-4 and H-5 Would allow Mike to continue on his schedule of three hospitalizations every two years without improvement of quality of life or measures to curtail the advance of the disease.

	Possible	My Score
H-1	- 1	
H-2	+ 3	+3
H-3	- 3	
H-4	- 3	
H-5	- 3	
Total	+ 3	+3

MIKE KOWALSKI

Route Section	Scoring: Possible	Scoring: My Score
A	16	17
D	3	3
C	3	3
F	2	
B	10	5
E	21	21
G	3	3
K	11	9
J	3	3
II	3	3
TOTAL	73	67

(Route: A → D → C → B, with an alternate branch C → F → B; then B → E → G → K → J → II)

Optimal Route Passing Score <u>50</u>
Alternate Route CFB Passing Score <u>51</u>

REFERENCES

1. Burton Hodgkins: **Respiratory Care, a Guide to Clinical Practice, 2nd Edition,** Lippincott, 1984. (Pages 282-297, 438, 456-489, 656-676, 678-693).

2. Mitchell & Petty: **Synopsis of Clinical Pulmonary Disease, 3rd Edition,** C. V. Mosby, 1982. (Pages 97-112).

3. O'Ryan: **Pulmonary Rehabilitation from Hospital to Home,** Yearbook Medical Publishers, 1984. (Pages 64-81).

4. Shapiro: **Clinical Application of Respiratory Care, 3rd Edition,** Year Book Medical Publishers, 1985. (Pages 62-68, 76-77, 110-122, 133-134, 176-188).

Cliff Chambers
Clinical Simulation #2

Problem

CLIFF CHAMBERS

You are a staff respiratory therapist on the day shift of a 250-bed religious order hospital. You are paged to the emergency room to participate in the care of Mr. Chambers.

The duty physician is busy with another emergency. He asks you to perform a preliminary pulmonary evaluation in his absence.

Mr. Chambers is 66 years old, has a past history of congestive heart failure and COPD. His chief complaint is severe shortness of breath. His medical history is one of three hospitalizations in the past two years—all pulmonary in nature.

NOW GO TO SECTION A

SECTION A

Which would you choose to evaluate?

Choose as many as you feel are indicated in this section.

A-1 Pupil reactivity	
A-2 Respiratory rate and pattern	22/min., I:E ratio 1:4, purse-lipped**
A-3 Accessory muscle use	Present**
A-4 Range of motion	
A-5 Temperature	38.9 C (102.8 F)**
A-6 Gag reflex	
A-7 Bowel sounds	
A-8 Pulse and blood pressure	108/min., 145/97 mmHg**
A-9 Hering-Breuer reflex	
A-10 Lower extremeties	Edematous feet and ankles**
A-11 Home medications	Ventolin Inhaler, Theo-dur tablets, "water" pills, digoxin**
A-12 Breath sounds	Diminished, end expiratory wheezing**

A-13 Posture	
A-14 Deep tendon reflex	
A-15 Diagnostic chest percussion	Dull, RLL; hyperresonant elsewhere, unequal diaphragmatic movement**
A-16 Chest inspection	Limited movement of costal margins, "barrel-shaped"**
A-17 Sputum	Small amount, thick, yellow, purulent**
A-18 Skin and mucus membranes	Diaphoretic, slight cyanosis lips and mouth**
A-19 Heart sounds	
When you have completed your selections in this section, then develop A-20	Go to Section N**

(R) lower Lobe Pneum.

SECTION B

An arterial blood gas is drawn 20 minutes after instituting mechanical ventilation. Results are pH 7.42, PCO_2 39 mmHg, PO_2 85 mmHg, HCO_3^-/25 mEq/l.

What ventilator changes would you recommend?

Choose only one, unless you are directed to "make another selection in this section."

B-1 Set PEEP at 5 cm H_2O	Physician disagrees, make another selection in this section.**
B-2 Set tidal volume at 800 ml	Physician agrees, tidal volume is reduced to 800 ml., go to Section C**
B-3 Set ventilator rate at 10/min.	Physician disagrees, make another selection in this section.**
B-4 Maintain present settings	Physician disagrees, make another selection in this section.**
B-5 Reduce ventilator rate to 6/min.	

SECTION C

Based on the results of your evaluation, what would you recommend?

Choose only one, unless you are directed to "make another selection in this section."

C-1 Add 5 cm H_2O PEEP

C-2 Increase rate to 10/min.

C-3 Increase FIO_2 to 0.5

C-4 Increase tidal volume to 1000 ml

C-5 Commence weaning procedures

End of problem**

SECTION D

The patient is transferred to the hospital's pulmonary service. Mr. Chambers' respiratory rate is 20/min., pulse is 94/min. The attending physician asks for your suggestions on orders to further treat the patient's respiratory condition.

Choose as many as you feel are indicated in this section.

D-1 Diaphragmatic breathing

D-2 Bronchodilator therapy

D-3 Hyperinflation therapy (IPPB with normal salinc)

D-4 Refer to the hospital's hyperbaric oxygen service

D-5 Incentive spirometry

D-6 Continuous ultrasonic nebulizer therapy

D-7 Cromolyn sodium administration

D-8 Pulmonary stress testing

D-9 Mask CPAP

D-10 Chest physical therapy

When you have completed your selections in this section, then develop D-11

SECTION E

Which tests would you request?

Choose as many as you feel are indicated in this section.

E-1 Bronchoscopy	
E-2 Complete blood count (CBC)	Hb 16 gm/100 ml, WBC 14,000/mm^3, elevated neutrophil count**
E-3 Ventilation/perfusion scan	
E-4 Serum electrolytes	Cl 104 mEq/l, Na 142 mEq/l, HCO_3 32 mEq/l, K 4.2 mEq/l**
E-5 D_LCO	
E-6 Sputum for gram stain and culture/sensitivity	Done, sample sent to laboratory**
E-7 P-50 (Measured)	
E-8 Chest x-ray	Density, RLL; evidence of hyperinflation**
E-9 ECG (12 lead)	Sinus tachycardia, rate 108/min., scattered multifocal PVC's**
E-10 Cardiac output	
E-11 V_d/V_t (% of deadspace)	
E-12 $C(a\text{-}v)_{02}$	
E-13 Cardiac enzymes	
E-14 Pulmonary capillary wedge	
E-15 Arterial blood gases	pH 7.31, PCO_2 60 mmHg, PO_2 52 mmHg, HCO_3 32 mEq/l**
E-16 FEV_{1sec}/FVC %	
	Go to Section D**

When you have completed your selections in this section, then develop E-16

SECTION F

Which tests would you request?

Choose as many as you feel are indicated in this section.

F-1 Bronchoscopy

F-2 Complete blood count (CBC) and differential

F-3 Ventilation/perfusion scan

F-4 Serum electrolytes

F-5 D_LCO

F-6 Sputum for gram stain and culture sensitivity

F-7 P-50 (Measured)

F-8 Chest x-ray

F-9 ECG (12 Lead)

F-10 Cardiac output

F-11 V_d/V_t (% of deadspace)

F-12 $(Ca - v)_{02}$

F-13 Cardiac enzymes

F-14 Pulmonary capillary wedge pressure

F-15 Arterial blood gases

F-16 FEV_{1sec}/FVC %

When you have completed your selections in this section, then develop F-17

SECTION G

After reporting your findings to the physician, he requests you obtain a stat arterial blood gas. He states he will be at the hospital as soon as possible.

Results of the arterial blood gas are pH 7.29, PCO_2 64 mmHg, PO_2 40 mmHg, HCO_3^- 34 mEq/l.

On the basis of these results, what will you recommend to the physician upon his arrival?

Choose only one, unless you are directed to "make another selection in this section."

G-1 Transfer to intensive care, intubate, institute CPAP 5 cm H_2O

G-2 Transfer to intensive care, intubate and mechanically ventilate

Physician agrees, go to Section H**

G-3 Intubate immediately, support ventilation via resuscitation bag FIO_2 0.80

G-4 Increase frequency of chest physical therapy to Q1°

G-5 Administer IPPB with 0.5 ml metaproternal and 2 ml normal saline Q4°

SECTION H

Which of the following ventilator modes would you recommend? Mr. Chambers is 5'10" (180 cm) and weighs 160 lbs. (73 kg).

Choose only one, unless you are directed to "make another selection in this section."

H-1 Assist control, FIO_2 1.0, rate 18, tidal volume 600 ml

H-2 Assist control mode FIO_2 0.4, rate 8, tidal volume 1,000 ml

H-3 IMV mode, FIO_2 0.4, rate 4, tidal volume 1,000 ml

H-4 IMV mode, FIO_2 0.4, Rate 8, tidal volume 1,000 ml

H-5 Control mode, FIO_2 0.6, rate 16, tidal volume 900 ml

SECTION I

Which of the following oxygen administration devices would you recommend to initiate therapy?

Choose only one, unless you are directed to "make another selection in this section."

I-1 A 40% venturi mask

I-2 A simple mask at 2 L/min.

I-3 A nasal cannula at 2 L/min.

I-4 A partial rebreather mask

I-5 A non-rebreather mask

SECTION J

The next day you see Mr. Chambers while doing your oxygen rounds. He fails to respond to your greeting and answers your questions inappropriately. Prior to calling his attending physician, which would you choose to properly and quickly assess the patient's respiratory status?

Choose as many as you feel are indicated in this section.

J-1 Gag reflex	
J-2 Tidal volume	
J-3 Vital capacity	
J-4 Negative inspiratory force	Unable to perform**
J-5 Breath sounds	Diffuse expiratory wheezing; diminished right and left lower lobes, some crackles**
J-6 Respiratory rate and pattern	32/min, intercostal and supra-clavicular retractions**
J-7 Babinski reflex	
J-8 Orientation to time and place	Disoriented**
J-9 Deep tendon reflex	
J-10 Temperature and pulse	103 F, 124/min.**
J-11 Pulmonary compliance	
When you have completed your selections in this section, then develop J-12	Go to Section G**

SECTION K

Based on information you now have, which would be your recommendation as to the first course of action in Mr. Chambers' treatment?

Choose only one, unless you are directed to "make another selection in this section."

K-1 Perform pulmonary function studies

K-2 Commence oxygen therapy

K-3 Commence bronchodilator therapy

K-4 Assist ventilation via resuscitation bag

K-5 Intubate and support ventilation via resuscitation bag

SECTION L

Thirty minutes after arrival in the intensive care unit and institution of therapy, Mr. Chambers' arterial blood gases are as follows: pH 7.28, PCO_2 64 mmHg, PO_2 52 mmHg, HCO_3^- 30 mEq/l.

What would you recommend now?

Choose only one, unless you are directed to "make another selection in this section."

L-1 Mechanically ventilate

L-2 Increase CPAP to 10 cm H_2O

L-3 Continue present therapy monitor

L-4 Obtain serum electrolytes

L-5 Obtain cardiac enzymes

SECTION M

An arterial blood gas is ordered. It returns 10 minutes later with the following results: pH 7.31, PCO_2 58 mmHg, PO_2 62 mmHg, HCO_3^- 30 mEq/l. Cliff states he "is breathing much easier". What would you recommend now?

Choose only one, unless you are directed to "make another selection in this section."

M-1 Intubate and ventilate	
M-2 Order diagnostic procedures and laboratory tests	Physician agrees, go to Section E**
M-3 Administer aminophylline intravenously	
M-4 Administer 20% acetylcysteine via hand held nebulizer	
M-5 Support ventilation via resuscitation bag	

SECTION N

Based on your assessment, which would be your recommendation as to the first course of action in Mr. Chambers' treatment?

Choose only one, unless you are directed to "make another selection in this section."

N-1 Perform pulmonary function studies

N-2 Commence oxygen therapy

N-3 Commence bronchodilator therapy

N-4 Assist ventilation via resuscitation bag

N-5 Order further diagnostic tests

SECTION O

48 Hours later, the patient has stabilized. You are asked to re-evaluate his cardiopulmonary status.

Which would you choose?

Choose as many as you feel are indicated in this section.

O-1 Pulmonary artery pressure	
O-2 Static compliance	42 ml/cm H_2O**
O-3 Colloid osmotic pressure	
O-4 Chest x-ray	Endotracheal tube in place, evidence of hyperinflation**
O-5 % Shunt (Q_s/Q_t) estimated	
O-6 Serum electrolytes	Cl 104 mEq/l, Na 143 mEq/l, HCO_3 29 mEq/l, K+ 4.2 mEq/l**
O-7 V_d/V_t (% of deadspace)	
O-8 P-50 measured	
O-9 Vital capacity	1.8 litres**
O-10 Spontaneous tidal volume and rate	420 ml, 12/min.**
O-11 Lung diffusion test (D_LCO)	
O-12 Mixed venous PO_2	
O-13 Carboxyhemoglobin	
O-14 Arterial blood gases	pH 7.39, PCO_2 52 mmHg, PO_2 66 mmHg, HCO_3 29 mEq/l**
O-15 Negative inspiratory force	-28 cm H_2O**
O-16 Electrocardiogram	Sinus rhythm, rate 90/min., scattered PVC's**
O-17 When you have completed your selections in this section, then develop O-17	Go to Section C**

SECTION P

Which would you recommend?

Choose only one, unless you are directed to "make another selection in this section."

P-1 A 28% venturi mask

P-2 A 40% venturi mask

P-3 An O_2 mask at 2 l/p/m

P-4 A partial rebreather mask (flow sufficient to prevent the bag from collapsing)

P-5 A nasal cannula at 6 l/p/m

P-6 A nasal cannula at 2 l/p/m

Cliff Chambers
Clinical Simulation #2

Answers,
Explanations,
and Scoring

CLIFF CHAMBERS

This problem centers on a COPD patient. Central to his management is recognition of "normal" arterial blood gases, criteria for ventilator commitment, ventilator management, and weaning criteria.

SECTION A

Positive Scoring:

A-2, A-3, A-12, A-13, A-15, A-16, A-17, and A-18 Are basic elements of a pulmonary evaluation that may be performed without resorting to specific testing. They are rapidly assessed and are accepted indicators of pulmonary status, when performed by a knowledgeable therapist.

A-5, A-8, A-10, and A-11 Are evaluations important, but peripheral to pulmonary assessment — hence, scored at a lesser value.

Negative Scoring:

A-1 Pupil reactivity is irrelevant in a patient described in the scenario.

A-4 Range of motion is not a factor in a pulmonary assessment.

A-6 The patient's ability to swallow is not in question.

A-7 Is outside the scope of a pulmonary assessment.

A-14 Is unnecessary and cruel.

A-19 Is also outside the scope of a pulmonary assessment.

	Possible	My Score
A-1	- 1	
A-2	+2	+2
A-3	+2	+2
A-4	- 2	
A-5	+1	+1
A-6	- 2	
A-7	- 2	
A-8	+1	+1
A-9	- 2	
A-10	+1	+1
A-11	+1	+1
A-12	+2	+2
A-13	+2	+2
A-14	- 2	
A-15	+2	+2
A-16	+1	+1
A-17	+2	+2
A-18	+2	+2
A-19	- 2	
Total	**19**	19

SECTION N

Positive Scoring:

N-2 From your assessment, it should be apparent our patient is a CHF/COPD in an acute episode of pulmonary infection. This is evident from temperature, sputum, respiratory rate, etc. The fact there is some cyanosis mandates the administration of oxygen immediately.

N-5 More definitive studies are needed prior to commencement of treatment. There are many unanswered questions. To deny Mr. Chambers some relief for his shortness of breath while awaiting results would do him a disservice. For choosing this option you are awarded lesser points and diverted to an alternate route.

Negative Scoring:

N-1 Would be of no immediate benefit.

N-3 In view of the fact the patient is in a state of hypoxia/hypoxemia, this might not be effective. We really don't know if bronchospasm is a component of the problem.

N-4 We have not established adequacy or inadequacy of ventilation as the cause of hypoxia. It is not a realistic means of relieving Cliff's dyspnea.

	Possible	My Score
N-1	- 3	
N-2	+ 3	+3
N-3	- 3	
N-4	- 3	
N-5	+ 1	
Total	**+ 3**	+3

ALTERNATE ROUTE

SECTION F

Positive Scoring:

F-6, F-8, F-15, and F-16 Are tests central to pinpointing the underlying cause, and its severity.

F-2 and F-9 Would yield information of definite value, but still peripheral to treating or diagnosing the patient's chief complaint.

Zero Scoring:

F-4 Although electrolytes are somewhat redundant, they do verify the patient's metabolic compensation for an underlying, chronic, respiratory acidosis. (HCO_3^- 30 meQ/l) This is a measured value (not calculated), hence very reliable.

Negative Scoring:

F-1, F-3, F-5, F-7, F-10, F-11, F-12, and F-14 Are all tests which would require catheterization and instrumentation which are not emergency room procedures.

F-13 There is no evidence of myocardial infection. The test would be redundant.

	Possible	My Score
F-1	- 2	
F-2	+ 1	
F-3	- 2	
F-4	0	
F-5	- 2	
F-6	+ 2	
F-7	- 2	
F-8	+ 2	
F-9	+ 1	
F-10	- 1	
F-11	- 1	
F-12	- 2	
F-13	- 1	
F-14	- 1	
F-15	+ 2	
F-16	+ 2	
Total	**10**	

SECTION I

Positive Scoring:

I-3 This is a standard order for a suspected carbon dioxide retainer. It is safe in that it avoids any risk of oxygen induced hypoventilation—as documented in the literature. Two liters per minute via nasal cannula equates to an FIO_2 of 0.28.

Negative Scoring:

I-1 Exceeds the acceptable FIO_2 as an initial order on a COPD of unknown response to supplemental oxygen therapy.

I-2 Is contraindicated. 2 Liters per minute is insufficient to flush carbon dioxide from a mask.

I-4 and I-5 Also exceed safe limits with 60-90% and 100% respectively.

	Possible	My Score
I-1	- 3	
I-2	- 3	
I-3	+ 3	+3
I-4	- 3	
I-5	- 3	
Total	**+ 3**	+3

ALTERNATE ROUTE

SECTION K

Positive Scoring:

K-2 The data documents the fact that the patient is a COPD patient with some underlying cardiac involvement, with acidosis, hypoxia, and infection. He will require hospitalization of some duration.

Prior to his transfer to the pulmonary service, oxygen therapy will alleviate his shortness of breath—the chief complaint.

Negative Scoring:

K-1 Is clinically unrealistic. The information may be helpful but not at this point.

K-3 Is not indicated. We don't know if bronchospasm is a component of the problem.

K-4 Is unrealistic in that the arterial blood gases indicate some reserve, if the oxygenation status can be improved by supplemental oxygen.

K-5 as in K-4 This move would be premature prior to oxygen therapy.

	Possible	My Score
K-1	- 3	
K-2	+ 3	
K-3	- 3	
K-4	- 3	
K-5	- 3	
Total	+ 3	

SECTION M

Positive Scoring:

M-2 The patient has responded to supplemental oxygen therapy. More information is needed to commence specific therapies. The immediate problem has been addressed and this action now becomes the priority.

Negative Scoring:

M-1 Is not indicated. The blood gas results must be interpreted in light of the patient's preexisting pulmonary disease. A typical blood gas of a patient with similar symptomology, under normal circumstances is approximately pH 7.34, PCO_2 55, PO_2 55, HCO_3^- 29.

M-3 The patient's response to aerosolized bronchodilators is not yet established. This course of action could be redundant. It would be premature.

M-4 There is no evidence that removal of secretions is a problem.

M-5 The patient's dyspnea is sufficient, as evidenced by his statement. No support is needed.

	Possible	My Score
M-1	- 3	
M-2	+ 3	+3
M-3	- 3	
M-4	- 3	
M-5	- 3	
Total	**+ 3**	+3

SECTION P

Positive Scoring:

P-3 This is a standard order for a suspected carbon dioxide retainer. It is safe in that it avoids any risk of oxygen induced hypoventilation—as documented in the literature. Two liters per minute via nasal cannula equates to an FIO_2 of 0.28.

P-6 Is also a standard order in many hospitals, but because the FIO_2 is dependant on respiratory rate and title volume it is not the "best choice" for a CO_2 retainer.

Negative Scoring:

P-1 Exceeds the acceptable FIO_2 as an initial order on a COPD of unknown response to supplemental oxygen therapy.

P-2 Is contraindicated. 2 Liters per minute is insufficient to flush carbon dioxide from a mask.

P-4 and P-5 Also exceed safe limits with 60-90% and 100% respectively.

	Possible	My Score
P-1	- 3	
P-2	- 3	
P-3	+ 3	
P-4	- 3	
P-5	- 3	
P-6	+ 1	
Total	**3**	

SECTION E

Positive Scoring:

E-6, E-8, E-15, and E-16 Are tests central to pinpointing the underlying cause, and its severity.

E-2 and E-9 Would yield information of definite value, but still peripheral to treating or diagnosing the patient's chief complaint.

Zero Scoring:

E-4 Although electrolytes are somewhat redundant, they do verify the patient's metabolic compensation for an underlying, chronic, respiratory acidosis. (HCO_3^- 30 mEq/l) This is a measured value (not calculated) — hence very reliable.

Negative Scoring:

E-1, E-3, E-5, E-7, E-10, E-11, E-12, and E-14 Are all tests which would require catheterization and instrumentation which are not emergency room procedures.

E-13 There is no evidence of myocardial infarction. The test would be redundant.

	Possible	My Score
E-1	- 2	
E-2	+ 1	+1
E-3	- 2	
E-4	0	0
E-5	- 2	
E-6	+ 2	+2
E-7	- 2	
E-8	+ 2	+2
E-9	+ 1	+1
E-10	- 1	
E-11	- 1	
E-12	- 2	
E-13	- 1	
E-14	- 1	
E-15	+ 2	+2
E-16	+ 2	
Total	**10**	8

SECTION D

Positive Scoring:

D-2 Bronchodilator therapy would now be indicated on a trial basis.

D-10 Chest physical therapy would be useful adjunctive therapy to aid removal of secretions.

Zero Scoring:

D-3 The controversial and regional aspects of this therapy mandates zero scoring. Theoretically it might be of value. However, prevalent thought and practice relegates this modality to the patient who is unable, or refuses, to take a deep breath.

Negative Scoring:

D-1 Is a rehabilitation procedure.

D-4 There are no indications present for HBO.

D-5 Is indicated exclusively for the post-operative patient.

D-6 There is no evidence water needs to be added to the airways.

D-7 Is a prophylactic anti-asthmatic drug.

D-8 Is not indicated in the patient's acute condition.

D-9 The patient's oxygenation status is not precipitous or refractory.

	Possible	My Score
D-1	- 2	-2
D-2	+2	+2
D-3	0	
D-4	- 2	
D-5	- 1	
D-6	- 1	
D-7	- 2	
D-8	- 2	
D-9	- 2	
D-10	+2	+2
Total	**4**	+2

SECTION J

Positive Scoring:

Prior to informing a physician one of his patients has deteriorated, it is prudent to be prepared with facts.

J-5, J-6, J-8, and J-10 Are solid evidence to validate your call.

Zero Scoring:

J-2 Your practice of respiratory care may or may not encompass carrying a volumetric measuring device in your pocket (Wright Respirometer, Bournes LS 75, etc.) — hence no penalty; although it would be useful information.

Negative Scoring:

J-1, J-7, J-18, and J-9 Are tests to assess neurologic function in the comatose patient, exclusively.

J-3 and J-4 Specialized equipment is needed, and not available.

J-11 For all practical purposes, is only available on an intubated patient.

	Possible	My Score
J-1	- 2	
J-2	0	
J-3	- 1	
J-4	- 2	
J-5	+2	+2
J-6	+2	+2
J-7	- 2	
J-8	+2	+2
J-9	- 2	
J-10	+2	+2
J-11	- 2	
Total	**8**	8

SECTION G

Positive Scoring:

G-1 CPAP assumes the oxygenation status of the patient is due to shunt only. This may or may not be the case, but is a possibility. It only addresses the problem of oxygenation. The acid base patient status would be unresolved. Transferring the patient to an intensive care makes this response forgiveable.

G-2 The blood gas results depict a patient in acute respiratory failure. The indicators are present to intubate and ventilate. This is the preferable response. This mandates transfer to an intensive care unit.

Negative Scoring:

G-3 This should only be done where intensive care facilities are unavailable, and won't be available for some time.

G-4 More vigorous removal of secretions by this time consuming modality would ignore the serious, acute status of the patient.

G-5 As in G-4, the acute, serious nature of the patient's status is ignored.

	Possible	My Score
G-1	+ 1	
G-2	+ 3	+3
G-3	- 3	
G-4	- 3	
G-5	- 3	
Total	+ 3	+3

ALTERNATE ROUTE

SECTION L

Positive Scoring:

L-1 The patient has deteriorated, although his oxygenation status is improved somewhat. The acid-base status is precipitous and mechanical ventilation will be required to reverse this downward trend.

Negative Scoring:

L-2 and L-3 Have proven ineffective.

L-4 and L-5 Would accomplish nothing to reverse the downward spiral of the patient.

	Possible	My Score
L-1	+ 1	
L-2	- 3	
L-3	- 3	
L-4	- 3	
L-5	- 3	
Total	+ 1	

SECTION H

Positive Scoring:

H-2 and H-4 Are scored equally. Either mode is satisfactory for a spontaneously breathing patient. In each case, the criteria for initial tidal volume is met, (12-15 ml/kg), as is minute volume and safe dosage of supplemental oxygen (< 0.5).

Negative Scoring:

H-1 Does not meet initial tidal volume criteria. FIO_2 is excessive, and a minute volume of 10.8 liters is high.

H-3 Has insufficient ventilation and excessive FIO_2.

H-5 Is contraindicated for a non-apneic patient. FIO_2 Is excessive, as is respiratory rate.

	Possible	My Score
H-1	- 3	
H-2	+ 3	
H-3	- 3	
H-4	+ 3	+3
H-5	- 3	
Total	+ 3	+3

SECTION B

Positive Scoring:

B-2 and B-5 Individually, or together will effect the return to the patient's abnormal status (for him normal). Note the HCO_3^- of 25 mEq/l. This is incorrect as this value is calculated from the pH and PCO_2—not measured. By quickly reversing a compensated patient, they are left in a state of acute metabolic alkalosis. Serious consequences may arise from this situation.

Negative Scoring:

B-1 Is not indicated. PO_2 is not refractory.

B-3 Is moving in the wrong direction.

B-4 As explained above, for a compensated COPD patient, this is not a normal blood gas. A normal would be, approximately the values described in Section M.

	Possible	My Score
B-1	- 3	
B-2	+ 3	+3
B-3	- 3	
B-4	- 3	-3
B-5	+ 3	
Total	+ 3	0

SECTION O

Positive Scoring:

At this point, and with the information that Cliff has "stabilized", it follows that a respiratory practitioner should be thinking "weaning". Given the severe hazards of mechanical ventilation, the sooner, the better. The criteria, as described on page 650 of Burton and Hodgkins have been sufficiently satisfied.

O-2 Is a satisfactory figure. It is somewhat high, but probably normal under the circumstances.

O-4 A clear chest x-ray indicates resolution of the basic pathology causing the hospitalization.

O-5, O-7, O-9, O-10, and O-15 All meet the criteria as per the reference above.

O-14 Indicates a return to normal.

O-16 Is precautionary. Presumably he is monitored and only requires a visual check.

Zero Scoring:

O-3 Could be of value, remotely in assessing risk of pleural effusion associated with CHF.

O-6 Is essentially redundant, but reaffirms Cliff's return to a normal compensated state (HCO_3^- 29 mEq/l).

Negative Scoring:

O-1 and O-12 Are unavailable as they require pulmonary artery catheterization.

O-11 Is not a weaning criteria.

O-8 and O-13 Hemoglobin abnormality is not in question.

	Possible	My Score
O-1	- 1	
O-2	+ 1	+1
O-3	0	
O-4	+ 2	+2
O-5	+ 2	
O-6	0	0
O-7	+ 1	
O-8	- 2	
O-9	+ 2	+2
O-10	+ 2	+2
O-11	- 2	
O-12	- 1	
O-13	- 2	
O-14	+ 2	+2
O-15	+ 2	+2
O-16	+ 1	+1
Total	**15**	12

SECTION C

Positive Scoring:

C-5 Weaning is indicated beyond doubt.

Negative Scoring:

C-1, C-2, C-3, and C-4 Would either be contraindicated (PEEP), or harmful (increased: rate, FIO_2, and tidal volume).

	Possible	My Score
C-1	- 3	
C-2	- 3	
C-3	- 3	
C-4	- 3	
C-5	+ 3	+3
Total	**+ 3**	+3

CLIFF CHAMBERS

ROUTE AND SCORING

ROUTE **SCORING**

ROUTE	Possible	My Score
A	19	19
N	3	3
F	10	
I	3	3
K	3	
M	3	3
P	3	
E	10	8
D	4	
J	8	8
G	3	3
L	1	
H	3	+3
B	3	0
O	15	12
C	3	+3
TOTAL	**77**	65

Optimal Route Passing Score **52**
All Alternate Routes **51**

REFERENCES

1. Burton, Hodgkins: **Respiratory Care a Guide to Clinical Practice, 2nd Edition,** Lippincott, 1984. (Pages 648-651)

2. Mitchell & Petty: **Synopsis of Clinical Pulmonary Disease, 3rd Edition,** C.V. Mosby, 1982. (Page 648-651)

3. Pilbeam: **Mechanical Ventilation Physiologic Applications and Clinical Applications,** Multi-Media Publishing, Inc., C.V. Mosby, 1986. (Pages 44-46, 53-60, 103-109, 163-205, 273-296)

4. Shapiro: **Clinical Application of Respiratory Care, 3rd Edition,** Year Book Medical Publishers, 1985. (Pages 76-77, 201, 379-407, 502-510)

April Smith

Clinical Simulation #3

Problem

APRIL SMITH

You are a night-shift respiratory therapist assigned to the area trauma center. Your hospital is an 850-bed teaching facility operating in conjunction with a medical school. At 1:30 a.m. April Smith arrives at the unit via EMT ambulance. She has suffered multiple trauma to the face, trunk, and lower extremities as the result of a one car crash. She is about 25 years old.

NOW GO TO SECTION A

SECTION A

The resident on duty requests you evaluate the pulmonary status of the patient while he supervises the care of the patient.

Which would you choose to evaluate?

Choose as many as you feel are indicated in this section.

A-1 Level of consciousness	Conscious but incoherent, random non-specific movement of body and extremities**
A-2 ECG	Sinus tachycardia. Monitor rate 132/minute**
A-3 General appearance	Pale, cool to touch, contusions on chest, open fracture, right femur blood loss apparent**
A-4 Respiratory rate and pattern	28/minute, shallow**
A-5 Bowel sounds	
A-6 Ability to swallow	
A-7 Chest movement	Paradoxic, right hemithorax**
A-8 Pulse, blood pressure	120/minute, 105/60 mmHg**
A-9 Negative inspiratory force	
A-10 Tidal volume	230 ml**
A-11 Diagnostic chest percussion	Dull, right hemithorax**
A-12 Vital capacity	Unable to perform**
A-13 $FEV_{1sec}/FVC\%$	
A-14 Chest auscultation	Breath sounds absent RLL, vesicular sounds left lung fields**
A-15 Babinski Reflex	
A-16 **When you have completed your selections in this section, then develop A-16**	Go to Section M**

SECTION B

Twenty four hours later, April's condition deteriorates. She is restless, agitated, and dusky. Data are:

ABG's: pH 7.34, PCO_2 49 mmHg, PO_2 46 mmHg, HCO_3^- 22 mEq/l

Hemodynamic data:

PCWP	16 mmHg
Cardiac output	6.8 L/min.
% shunt	38%
Blood pressure	115/68 mmHg
PAP	36/20 mmHg
$(Ca\text{-}Cv)_{02}$	2.3 vol%
PvO_2	32 mmHg

Ventilator Parameters:

Control mode	
PEEP	5 cm H_20
Rate	12/minute
FIO_2	0.4
Tidal volume	650 ml

Which would you recommend?

Choose only one, unless you are directed to "make another selection in this section."

B-1 Reduce rate to 6/minute and tidal volume to 600 ml

B-2 Increase PEEP after performing "Best" PEEP study

B-3 Diurese the patient

B-4 Increase volume of infused fluid

B-5 Increase FIO_2 to 0.60

Physician agrees, go to Section O**

SECTION C

To correct this problem, what would you recommend?

Choose only one, unless you are directed to "make another selection in this section."

C-1 Increase the high pressure Alarm setting 10 cm H_20	
C-2 Retract the endotracheal tube 2-4 cm	Physician agrees, go to Section E**
C-3 Request the resident to retract the endotracheal tube 2-4 cm	
C-4 Decrease the flow rate 5-10 liters/minute	Physician disagrees, make another selection in this section.**
C-5 Insert a chest tube. Right hemithorax	Physician disagrees, make another selection in this section.**

SECTION D

The resident asks your recommendations on tests/data which would aid in the treatment of April's respiratory problems. Which would you choose?

Choose as many as you feel are indicated in this section.

D-1 Bronchogram	
D-2 Carboxyhemoglobin level	
D-3 Hemoglobin/hematocrit	Hb 9.4 gm%, Hct 32.5%*
D-4 Chest x-ray	Done. Compound rib fractures, 2nd, 3rd, 4th, and 5th right ribs. Evidence of right lung contusion**
D-5 Neck x-ray	Cervical vertebrae intact**
D-6 Static compliance	
D-7 Lactic acid level	
D-8 12 lead ECG	Sinus tachycardia. Rate 112/min.*
D-9 Serum electrolytes	
D-10 P-50, measured	
D-11 Arterial blood gases	PH 7.30, PCO_2 52 mmHg, PO_2 48 mmHg, HCO_3^- 23.5 mEq/l, O_2 sat. 80%**
D-12 Venous O_2% satuation	
D-13 Urine pH	
D-14 Urine output	
D-15 **When you have completed your selections in this section, then develop D-15**	Go to Section P**

SECTION E

Static compliance is computed as follows:

PEEP	Static Compliance
7 1/2 cm H_20	28 ml/cm H_20
10 cm H_20	31 ml/cm H_20
12 1/2 cm H_20	37 ml/cm H_20
15 cm H_20	32 ml/cm H_20

Which PEEP setting would you choose?

Choose only one, unless you are directed to "make another selection in this section."

E-1 7 1/2 cm H_20

E-2 10 cm H_20

E-3 12 1/2 cm H_20

E-4 15 cm H_20

SECTION F

The patient is heavily sedated with valium and morphine. What ventilator parameters would you recommend? The patient weighs 110 lbs. (50 kg).

Choose only one, unless you are directed to "make another selection in this section."

F-1 Control mode, FIO_2 0.4, tidal volume 700 ml, rate 10/min., 5 cm H_20 PEEP

F-2 Control mode, FIO_2 0.4, Tidal volume 500 ml, rate 10/min., 5 cm H_20 PEEP

Done. 15 minutes later, ABG's pH 7.39, PCO_2 40 mm Hg, PO_2 80 mmHg, HCO_3^- 24 mEq/l, go to Section H.

F-3 Assist/control FIO_2 0.60, Tidal volume 500 ml, rate 10/min.

F-4 IMV, FIO_2 0.60, Tidal volume 500 ml, rate 10

F-5 Pressure support with 7 cm H_2O

SECTION G

To monitor the effects of the increased PEEP, which would you assess?

Choose as many as you feel are indicated in this section.

G-1 Complete blood count

G-2 ECG

G-3 Pulmonary artery pressure

G-4 PCWP

G-5 Cardiac output

G-6 Arterial blood gases

G-7 Central venous pressure

G-8 Mixed venous PO_2

G-9 Qs/Qt (% shunt measured)

G-10 Pulse, blood pressure

G-11 Serum electrolytes

G-12 Temperature

G-13 Ventilation/perfusion scan

G-14 **When you have completed your selections in this section, then develop G-14**

SECTION H

What would you recommend now?

Choose only one, unless you are directed to "make another selection in this section."

H-1 Increase tidal volume to 700 ml

H-2 Increase FIO_2 to 0.60

H-3 Increase rate to 14/minute

H-4 Maintain present ventilator settings. Re-evaluate in 30 minutes

H-5 Increase PEEP to 10 cm/H_20

SECTION I

After positioning the patient for the first chest physical therapy treatment, the ventilator high pressure sounds on each breath. To determine the cause, which would you evaluate?

Choose as many as you feel are indicated in this section.

I-1 Range of motion	
I-2 Patency of endotracheal tube	
I-3 Vital capacity	
I-4 FEV_{1sec}/FVC %	
I-5 Ventilator settings	
I-6 Ventilator circuitry	
I-7 Breath sounds	
I-8 Resistance to manual ventilation	
I-9 Ventilator pressure manometer reading	
I-10 Chest inspection	
I-11 Hering-Breuer reflex	
I-12 Negative inspiratory force	
I-13 Skin color	
I-14 Patient's sensorium	
I-15 Pupil reactivity	
I-16 Muscle strength	
I-17 **When you have completed your selections in this section, then develop I-17**	

SECTION J

At the conclusion of your shift, the resident on duty asks your opinion as to changes needed on ventilator parameters. Of the following, which would you suggest?

Ventilatory and hemodynamic data are unchanged.

Choose only one, unless you are directed to "make another selection in this section."

J-1 Increase PEEP to 15 cm H_2O	
J-2 Increase FIO_2	
J-3 Decrease rate to 6/minute, decrease tidal volume to 600 ml	
J-4 Start weaning procedures	Physician agrees, end of problem
J-5 Administer chronotropic and inatropic cardiac drugs	

SECTION K

Static compliance is computed as follows:

PEEP	Static Compliance
7 1/2 cm H_20	28 ml/cm H_20
10 cm H_20	31 ml/cm H_20
12 1/2 cm H_20	37 ml/cm H_20
15 cm H_20	32 ml/cm H_20

Which PEEP setting would you choose?

Choose only one, unless you are directed to "make another selection in this section."

K-1 7 1/2 cm H_20

K-2 10 cm H_20

K-3 12 1/2 cm H_20

K-4 15 cm H_20

SECTION L

Twenty four hours later, April's condition has stabilized. She has undergone surgery, has appropriate antibiotic therapy underway, as well as other indicated advanced cardiac life support measures. Data are:

ABG's: pH 7.44, PCO_2 37 mmHg, PO_2 85 mmHg, HCO_3^- 24 mEq/l

X-Ray report: RML atelectasis, increased since last report. Endotracheal tube 2 cm above the carina. Pulmonary artery catheter in place. Rib fractures, rt. 2nd, 3rd, 4th, and 5th ribs reduced and healing.

What would be your recommendation at this time?

Choose only one, unless you are directed to "make another selection in this section."

L-1 Maintain present ventilator Parameters. Monitor vital signs	
L-2 Increase tidal volume to 800 ml	
L-3 Increase FIO_2 to 0.5	
L-4 Raise PEEP to 10 cm H_2O	Physician disagrees, make another selection in this section.**
L-5 Perform postural drainage, right middle lobe	Physician agrees, go to Section I**

SECTION M

On the basis of the information you have, which course of action would you recommend to follow immediately?

Choose only one, unless you are directed to "make another selection in this section."

M-1 Intubate and place on CPAP. 5 Cm H_20, FIO_2 0.4	Physician disagrees, make another selection in this section.**
M-2 Intubate and mechanically ventilate	Physician disagrees, make another selection in this section.**
M-3 Administer oxygen via a 40% venturi mask	Done. Go to Section D**
M-4 Obtain chest x-rays	Physician disagrees, make another selection in this section.**
M-5 Transport to radiology department for computerized analogue tomography (CAT) scan	Physician disagrees, make another selection in this section.**

SECTION O

Fifteen minutes later arterial blood gases are: pH 7.45, PCO_2 35 mmHg, PO_2 48 mmHg, HCO_3^- 22 meQ/l. The hemodynamic data remains unchanged.

What would you recommend now?

Choose only one, unless you are directed to "make another selection in this section."

O-1 Perform "Fluid Challenge" procedure	
O-2 Perform therapeutic Bronchoscopy	
O-3 Decrease volume of infused fluid	
O-4 Increase FIO_2 to 0.8	
O-5 Increase PEEP after performing "Best PEEP" study	Physician agrees: go to Section K**

SECTION P

From the information gathered, what would you recommend as to the patients ongoing treatment?

Choose only one, unless you are directed to "make another selection in this section."

P-1	Intubate and mechanically ventilate	Physician agrees, go to Section F**
P-2	Assist ventilation via resuscitation bag FIO_2 0.4	Physician disagrees, make another selection in this section.**
P-3	Oxygen and aerosol therapy via face tent, FIO_2 0.4	
P-4	Intubate, administrate CPAP, 10 cm H_2O, FIO_2 0.4	
P-5	Bronchodilator therapy albuterol 2.5 mg via hand held nebulizer	

SECTION Q

Fifteen minutes after institution of CPAP, arterial blood gases are 7.29, PCO_2 56 mmHg, PO_2 48, HCO_3^- 22 meQ/l. Which would you recommend now?

Choose only one, unless you are directed to "make another selection in this section."

Q-1 Increase CPAP to 15 cm H_20

Q-2 Maintain present therapy, monitor

Q-3 Increase FIO_2 to 1.0

Q-4 Institute mechanical ventilation

Q-5 Sedate with valium and morphine

April Smith

Clinical Simulation #3

Answers, Explanations, and Scoring

APRIL SMITH

This problem requires management of trauma with concomitant flail chest. Pulmonary evaluation, ventilator commitment, solution of a right mainstem intubation problem, and "best" PEEP are integral components.

SECTION A

Positive Scoring:

A-4, A-7, A-10, A-11 and A-14 Are central elements of a pulmonary assessment.

A-1, A-2, A-3, and A-8 Are assessments of value, but not central to a "pulmonary" evaluation—hence, the lower scoring.

The information gathered, and the scenario, are typical of trauma cases. They are at risk to, flail chest, ARDS, blood loss, and with long bone breaks and fat emboli. When mechanically ventilated, they are subject to all these concomitant hazards.

Negative Scoring:

A-5 Bowel sounds are beyond the scope of a pulmonary evaluation.

A-6 and A-15 Applicable only with neurological disease or deep coma.

A-9 Is inappropriate with a patient of this category. It is a weaning procedure, primarily.

A-12 and A-13 Are effort dependent and inappropriate for a patient unable to follow commands.

	Possible	My Score
A-1	+1	+1
A-2	+1	+1
A-3	+1	+1
A-4	+2	+2
A-5	-2	
A-6	-2	
A-7	+2	+2
A-8	+1	+1
A-9	-1	
A-10	+2	+2
A-11	+2	+2
A-12	-1	-1
A-13	-1	
A-14	+2	+2
A-15	-2	
Total	**14**	13

SECTION M

Positive Scoring:

M-3 The initial evaluation describes a patient in shock which mandates immediate treatment with oxygen. The spectre of flail chest is equally indicative for immediate oxygen therapy. The patient probably is in a state of stagnant hypoxia (shock) and hypoxic hypoxia (hypoventilation).

Negative Scoring:

M-1 and M-2 We do not yet know if the indications exist for either of these actions. They probably are, but one not to be done "immediately".

M-4 and M-5 Are distinct possibilities, but, only after oxygen therapy is underway.

	Possible	My Score
M-1	- 3	
M-2	- 3	
M-3	+ 3	+3
M-4	- 3	
M-5	- 3	
Total	+ 3	+3

SECTION D

Positive Scoring:

D-3 Evidence of blood loss could be a factor in oxygen transport.

D-4 Is imperative. It alerts us to flail chest and its extent as well as lung parenchymal involvement.

D-5 Is a definite consideration as to how the patient is manipulated for respiratory procedures.

D-8 Is of peripheral importance to oxygenation.

D-11 Is of central importance in the patient's respiratory management. It verifies hypoxia and a serious, acute, respiratory situation.

Zero Scoring:

D-9 Could be of some value, but is not likely as the patient presumably, was in a healthy state prior to her crash.

Negative Scoring:

D-1 Is indicated for airways disease and bronchiectasis specifically.

D-2 Carbon monoxide status is not in question.

D-6 and D-12 Would require intubation and catheterization respectively.

D-7 Anoxia is not mentioned where metabolic acidosis could possibly be in question.

D-10 Hemoglobin abnormality is not in question.

D-13 and D-14 Are beyond the scope of ventilatory management of a trauma patient.

	Possible	My Score
D-1	-2	
D-2	-2	
D-3	+2	+2
D-4	+2	+2
D-5	+2	+2
D-6	-1	
D-7	-1	
D-8	+1	+1
D-9	0	
D-10	-2	
D-11	+2	+2
D-12	-1	
D-13	-2	
D-14	-2	
Total	**9**	9

SECTION P

Positive Scoring:

P-1 Is indicated by the clinical picture and the blood gases. Positive pressure is indicated to support the flailing chest as is mechanical ventilation to address the central problem of acute ventilatory failure.

P-4 Positive pressure in the form of CPAP is indicated to treat flail chest. It does not address the central problem. This choice takes you through an alternate route.

Negative Scoring:

P-2 Is only putting off the inevitable. At best, it is a temporary measure in the treatment of acute respiratory failure.

P-3 Is unacceptable as it ignores the need for effective ventilation.

P-5 Bronchoconstriction is not in question.

	Possible	My Score
P-1	+ 3	+3
P-2	- 3	-3
P-3	- 3	
P-4	+ 1	
P-5	- 3	
Total	+ 3	0

ALTERNATE ROUTE
SECTION Q

Positive Scoring:

Q-4 Is the obvious choice. The blood gases document the fact that a trial of CPAP was a failure. It did help the oxygenation status, somewhat, but the patient is still hypoventilating and in ventilatory failure.

Negative Scoring:

Q-1 CPAP has failed.

Q-2 Would continue the deteriorating status of the patient.

Q-3 Would not reverse ventilatory failure.

Q-5 Would hasten and abett ventilatory failure when used with CPAP — which relies on a spontaneously breathing patient.

	Possible	My Score
Q-1	- 3	
Q-2	- 3	
Q-3	- 3	
Q-4	+ 1	
Q-5	- 3	
Total	**+ 1**	

SECTION F

Positive Scoring:

F-1 A "heavily sedated" patient mandates the control mode. It also is a preferable situation to splint or stabilize a flail chest — as is PEEP. PEEP is indicated due to lung contusion (probable shunt) and the distinct possibility of the onset of ARDS. Calculation of initial tidal volume (12-15 ml/kg = 600-750 ml) makes this choice inclusive of a correct tidal volume.

F-2 Takes you on an alternate route, although, the blood gases depict an underventilated patient. You were on the proper course.

Negative Scoring:

F-3 and F-4 Both contain inadequate tidal volumes. PEEP is also absent.

F-5 Is strictly a weaning procedure.

	Possible	My Score
F-1	+ 3	
F-2	+ 1	+1
F-3	- 3	
F-4	- 3	
F-5	- 3	
Total	+ 3	+1

ALTERNATE ROUTE
SECTION H

Positive Scoring:

H-1 and H-3 Are choices which would result in reversal of hypoventilation.

V_E = 10 x 700 ml = 7.0 liters

V_E = 14 x 500 ml = 7.0 liters

Either one rewards you with a return to the main route.

Negative Scoring:

H-2, H-4, and H-5 do not address the problem of hypoventilation and acid/base balance.

	Possible	My Score
H-1	+ 1	+1
H-2	- 3	
H-3	+ 1	
H-4	- 3	
H-5	- 3	
Total	+ 1	+ 1

SECTION L

Positive Scoring:

L-5 Is indicated for re-expansion of the right middle lobe. Re-expansion of that lobe is essential to the well-being of the patient.

Negative Scoring:

L-1 Ignores the problem of atelectasis as do the remaining choices.

L-2 Would upset acid base balance.

L-3 Is an unsafe dosage in the presence of a relatively satisfactory P_aO_2.

L-4 Would entail further risk, unnecessarily, to positive pressure in the thorax.

	Possible	My Score
L-1	-3	
L-2	-3	
L-3	-3	
L-4	-3	-3
L-5	+ 3	+3
Total	**+ 3**	0

SECTION I

Positive Scoring:

An abrupt, sudden, increase in ventilating pressure should cause one to think "restriction to flow".

I-2, I-6, and I-8 Are all choices that should lead to the conclusion that the problem lies within the patient — not the ventilator.

I-7 and I-10 Indicate the tip of the endotracheal tube has migrated into the right mainstem branches.

I-13 and I-14 Are choices which indicate an episode of hypoxia and the seriousness of the situation.

I-9 Would indicate the episode is not an aberrant positioning of the tube cuff over the tip or random movement of mucus near or around the tip.

I-5 An unauthorized change of ventilator settings could be the cause.

Negative Scoring:

I-1 Is a physical therapy procedure. Vital capacity (I-3 liters), $FEV_{1sec.}$, (I-4) could in no way determine a cause of the alarm.

I-11, I-12, I-15 and I-16 Are also unrelated to any possible cause for high pressure alarm.

	Possible	My Score
I-1	- 2	
I-2	+ 2	+2
I-3	- 2	
I-4	- 2	
I-5	+ 2	+2
I-6	+ 2	+2
I-7	+ 1	+1
I-8	+ 2	+2
I-9	+ 1	+1
I-10	+ 1	+1
I-11	- 2	
I-12	- 2	
I-13	+ 1	+1
I-14	+ 1	+1
I-15	- 2	
I-16	- 2	
Total	**13**	13

SECTION C

Positive Scoring:

C-2 Retracting the endotracheal tube in the face of right mainstem intubation is within the scope of respiratory care practice. This is also true of securing, cleaning, and changing artificial airways.

C-3 Might be more appropriate for some hospitals—hence, a positive, but lesser score.

Negative Scoring:

C-1 Might silence the alarm. It would be disasterous for the patient.

C-4 Is of no value towards solution of the problem.

C-5 A right tension pneumothorax, if present, would present quite differently. The right lower lobe would be absent of breath sounds. There would be detectable mediastinal/tracheal shift away from the affected side.

	Possible	My Score
C-1	- 3	
C-2	+ 3	+3
C-3	+ 1	
C-4	- 3	-3
C-5	- 3	-3
Total	+ 3	-3

SECTION B

Positive Scoring:

B-2 Refractory P_aO_2 mandates a PEEP higher than is presently the case. The physiology of PEEP is to raise FRC, open more unventilated alveolar units, and make more area available for gas exchange. A "best" PEEP study is required prior to making the change.

Zero Scoring:

B-5 The increase in FIO_2 will help the low PO_2, but in view of the amount of shunt, an increase in PEEP would be more appropriate.

Negative Scoring:

B-1 Is an inappropriate choice of ventilator management in view of the blood gases and other data given.

A review of the hemodynamic data indicates satisfactory values for a critical patient. Pulmonary capillary wedge pressure is elevated somewhat. % Shunt is not precipitous, pulmonary artery pressure is elevated somewhat, also. Arterial-venous difference and mixed venous PO_2 are diminished, but still at a level that would assure tissue oxygenation. All values would be consistent with ARDS. Choosing B-3 and B-4 carry a penalty for these reasons.

If you missed this point, it would serve you well to check the hemodynamics normals on pp. 300-304 of Shapiro's Clinical Application of Respiratory Care (Third Edition).

	Possible	My Score
B-1	-3	
B-2	+3	
B-3	-3	
B-4	-3	
B-5	0	0
Total	**+3**	0

ALTERNATE ROUTE

SECTION O

Positive Scoring:

O-5 The increase in FIO_2 did not produce the expected increase in P_aO_2. The P_aO_2 is refractory. Shunt is evident. This is the classic indication for PEEP. A "Best" PEEP study is mandated to set the optional level.

Negative Scoring:

O-1 A fluid challenge test is done where hypovolemia is suspected. A nominal bolus of fluid is infused. Blood pressure and PCWP responses are noted. An increase from below normal values serves as a guide to achieve satisfactory fluid balance.

O-2 There is no evidence of excess mucus or plugging to warrant therapeutic bronchoscopy.

O-3 Hemodynamic data does not indicate fluid overload.

O-4 Increasing FIO_2 has already proven refractory P_aO_2.

	Possible	My Score
O-1	-3	
O-2	-3	
O-3	-3	
O-4	-3	
O-5	+1	+1
Total	+1	+1

ALTERNATE ROUTE

SECTION K

Positive Scoring:

K-3 Achieves the highest or "Best" PEEP it will achieve the optimum conditions for gas exchange at the alveolar level.

Negative Scoring:

The other options (K-1, K-2, and K-4) open smaller volume per cm $H_2 0$ then does K-

	Possible	My Score
K-1	-3	
K-2	-3	
K-3	+ 1	+1
K-4	-3	
Total	**+ 1**	+1

SECTION E

Positive Scoring:

E-3 Achieves the highest or "Best" PEEP. It will achieve the optimum conditions for gas exchange at the alveolar level.

Negative Scoring:

The other options (E-1, E-2, and E-4) open smaller volume per cm H_20 then does E-3.

	Possible	My Score
E-1	- 3	
E-2	- 3	
E-3	+ 1	
E-4	- 3	
Total	+ 1	

SECTION G

Positive Scoring:

The effects of PEEP are dual faceted. On the one side are the hazards of positive pressure in the thorax. Namely, these are decreased cardiac output with decreasing blood pressure and subsequent hypoxia on the positive side is increased $P_{a}o_{2}$. This makes G-5, G-10, and G-6 central to evaluation of increase PEEP.

Implementation of PEEP is to improve the oxygenation status of the patient via the mechanism of decreased shunt. This makes G-9 central to evaluation of improved shunt.

Secondary to improved oxygenation are G-2, G-3, G-4, G-7, and G-8.

Negative Scoring:

G-1, G-11 and G-12 Would not effect, or be effected by the effects of increased PEEP.

G-13 Is not only redundant, it would stress the patient as it requires transport to and from the nuclear medicine department.

	Possible	My Score
G-1	- 2	
G-2	+ 1	+1
G-3	+ 1	+1
G-4	+ 1	+1
G-5	+ 2	+2
G-6	+ 2	+2
G-7	+ 1	+1
G-8	+ 1	+1
G-9	+ 1	+1
G-10	+ 2	+2
G-11	- 1	-1
G-12	- 2	
G-13	- 2	
Total	**12**	11

SECTION J

Positive Scoring:

J-3 Is the preferable response. These changes will bring the arterial blood gases closer to normal.

J-4 Weaning is premature. Before weaning can be considered, the underlying cause of the intubation/ ventilation must be substantially resolved. That problem was hypoventilation due to flail chest, followed by a bout of ARDS. Data from the previous section would indicate ARDS to be improved, but not resolved. Flail chest of this magnitude usually requires five days of positive pressure "splinting" before the ribs can resume their normal role in lung mechanics. The time frame of ventilation is approximately 2 1/2 days. Because a gradual approach toward weaning might be feasible, this choice is acceptable — but at a lesser score.

Negative Scoring:

J-1 The P_aO_2 is acceptable in light of the clinical presentation of the patient.

J-2 Is an unacceptably high dosage.

J-5 Cardiac drug administration, other than those used in resuscitative situations is beyond the scope of respiratory practice.

	Possible	My Score
J-1	-3	
J-2	-3	
J-3	+3	
J-4	+2	+2
J-5	-3	
Total	+3	+2

APRIL SMITH

ROUTE AND SCORING

Route	Possible	My Score
A	14	13
M	3	3
D	9	9
P	3	0
Q	[1]	
F	3	1
H	[1]	1
L	3	0
I	13	13
C	3	-3
B	3	0
O	[1]	1
K	[1]	1
E	3	
G	12	11
J	3	2
Total	**72**	52

Optimal Route Passing Score **50**
All Alternate Routes **49**

APRIL SMITH

REFERENCES

1. Burton, Hodgkins: **Respiratory Care a Guide to Clinical Practice, 2nd Edition,** Lippincott, 1984. (Pages 335, 648-651)

2. Pilbeam: **Mechanical Ventilation Physiologic Applications and Clinical Applications,** Multi-Media Publishing, Inc., C.V. Mosby, 1986. (Pages 229-232, 241)

3. Shapiro: **Clinical Application of Respiratory Care, 3rd Edition,** Year Book Medical Publishers, 1985. (Pages 62-68, 76-79, 176-187, 313-325, 379-407, 408-439)

Kathy Pope

Clinical Simulation #4

Problem

KATHY POPE

You are a staff respiratory therapist in a 110-bed suburban for profit hospital. During report prior to commencing the p.m.shift you receive a call from the department's medical director. He states one of his patients, Kathy Pope, is on her way into the hospital. He has directed Kathy's mother to bring her directly to the emergency room. He will be delayed, slightly, but will be in as soon as possible. He requests you meet them and perform a preliminary respiratory evaluation.

NOW GO TO SECTION A

SECTION A

You meet Kathy and her mother and relay the Doctor's message. Kathy is in obvious respiratory distress. The mother says Kathy has had asthma since infancy and this is the worst attack she has ever had. Kathy is 13 years old.

Which would you choose to evaluate?

Choose as many as you feel are indicated in this section.

A-1 Past medical history

A-2 Blood pressure

A-3 Temperature

A-4 Arterial blood gases

A-5 Hb, Hematocrit

A-6 Pulse

A-7 sputum examination

A-8 urinalysis

A-9 chest X-Ray

A-10 gag reflex

A-11 respiratory rate and pattern

A-12 V_d/T_t (% of deadspace)

A-13 breath sounds

A-14 FEV_1/FVC %

A-15 tactile fremitus

A-16 P50 measured

A-17 chest inspection

A-18 Diagnostic chest percussion

A-19 **When you have completed your selections in this section, then develop A-19**

SECTION B

Kathy fails to improve despite appropriate bronchodilator, IV aminophylline, and corticosteroid therapy. The physician quiz's you on which tests/procedures/monitoring would be appropriate for Kathy's treatment plan. He will order these which are appropriate.

Which would you choose?

Select as many as you feel are indicated in this section.

B-1 blood culture

B-2 sputum for gram stain

B-3 temperature, pulse, respiration

B-4 transfer to the intensive care unit

B-5 bedside spirometry (tidal volume, vital capacity, and peak flow rate)

B-6 computerized analogue tomography (CAT scan)

B-7 V_d/T_t (% of deadspace)

B-8 arterial blood gases

B-9 serum electrolytes, daily

B-10 urine, pH

B-11 theophylline level

B-12 chest X-Ray

B-13 pulmonary artery catherization

B-14 pedal edema

B-15 diffusion of the lung (D_LCO)

B-16 **When you have completed your selections in this section, then develop A-19**

SECTION C

The department equipment storage area has several ventilators ready for service. To implement mechanical ventilation for Kathy, which would provide the capabilities most suitable for her condition?

Choose only one, unless you are directed to "make another selection in this section."

C-1 An MA-1 Bennett with bellows spirometer and external PEEP valve

C-2 A PR-2 Bennett equipped with a cascade humidifier and bellows spirometer.

C-3 A Bourns BEAR 2

C-4 A Bourns BP 200

C-5 A 7200 Puritan-Bennett

SECTION E

Upon arrival in the intensive care unit blood gases are obtained. Results are pH 7.28, PCO_2 51mmHg, PO_2 48mmHg, HCO_3 22 mEq/l.

What would you recommend?

Choose only one, unless you are directed to "make another selection in this section."

E-1 Incentive spirometry

E-2 Continue present therapy and monitor.

E-3 Institute continuous ultrasonic nebulization therapy

E-4 Intubate and mechanically ventilate

SECTION F

The physician arrives. After ordering intravenous aminophylline and solumedrol he asks for your recommendations on respiratory therapy procedures which would aid in the treatment of the patient.

Which would you suggest?

Choose only one, unless you are directed to "make another selection in this section."

F-1 intubate and mechanically ventilate

F-2 Oxygen and bronchodilator therapy

F-3 Hyperinflation therapy (IPPB) with a bronchodilator

F-4 Mask CPAP 5cm H_2O FIO_2 0.28

F-5 Continuous heated aerosol therapy

SECTION G

Kathy weighs 102 lbs. (46kg) and is 149 cm tall. Which of the following would you select to commence mechanical ventilation?

Choose only one, unless you directed to "make another selection in this section."

G-1 Assist/control, tidal volume 500 ml, rate 10, flow rate 40 L/min., FIO_2 0.40

G-2 Control mode, tidal volume 500 ml, rate 12, flow rate 25 L/min., FIO_2 0.40, sedation will be necessary

G-3 SIMV mode, tidal volume 400 ml, rate 6, flow rate 50 L/min., FIO_2 0.50,

G-4 Assist/control mode, tidal volume 400 ml, rate 8, flow rate 30 L/min, FIO_2 0.40, 5 cm H_2O, PEEP

G-5 Assist/control mode, tidal volume 700 ml, rate 4, flow rate 30 L/min., FIO_2 0.40. Inspiratory pause 0.5 sec.

SECTION H

Based on the information gained in the previous section, which would you recommend?

Choose only one, unless you are directed to "make another selection in this section."

H-1 Reinflate the right lung with positive pressure	
H-2 Retract the endotracheal tube 2-4 cm	
H-3 Request insertion of a chest tube, right hemithorax	
H-4 Extracorpreal membrane oxygenation	
H-5 Insert a 22 gauge needle, right hemithorax between 4th and 5th intercostal space	

SECTION I

Fifteen minutes after commencing mechanical ventilation Kathy is quite agitated. She is out of synchrony with the ventilator. The high pressure alarm sounds periodically as does the I:E ratio.Which would you recommend?

Choose only one, unless you are directed to "make another selection in this section."

I-1 Increase the flow rate to 40 lpm

I-2 Add inspiratory pause 0.5 seconds

I-3 Set FIO_2 at 0.80

I-4 Sedate the patient and reduce flow rate to 25 lpm,

I-5 Increase the tidal volume to 700 ml

SECTION J

The physician asks for specifics as to how you would like the order written to accomplish therapy.

Which would you specify?

Choose only one, unless you are directed to "make another selection in this section."

J-1 Oxygen via 40% Venturi mask, 0.5 ml-1.0% isoproternol solution with 2cc NS Q4 hours via hand held nebulizer

J-2 Oxygen via nasal cannula 4 lpm 0.5cc bronkosol-1.0% solution with 2cc NS via hand held nebulizer Q4 hours

J-3 Oxygen via 40% venturi mask, 1.0 ml albuterol-0.5% solution with 2cc NS via hand held nebulizer Q4 hours

J-4 Oxygen via simple mask 2 lpm 1.0 ml Albuterol-0.5% solution with 2 cc NS via hand held nebulizer Q4 hours

J-5 Aerosol mask with oxygen bled in 2 lpm 1.0 ml Albuterol-0.5% solution via hand held nebulizer Q2 hours

SECTION K

After ten breaths from the hand held nebulizer, Kathy experiences heart palpitations and tremors of her extremities.

What would you recommend now?

Choose only one, unless directed to "make another selection in this section."

K-1 Change medication to 3mg atropine via hand held nebulizer

K-2 Change medication to beclamethasone (vanceril) inhaler, 2 puffs QID

K-3 Change medication to cromolyn sodium spinhaler, 2 puffs QID

K-4 Change medication to 0.5 ml albuterol-0.5% solution

K-5 Continue treatment as ordered

SECTION L

Three minutes into the IPPB treatment, the patient's pulse is 122/minute. Her shortness of breath increases as her anxiety level raises. What would you do now?

Choose only one, unless you are directed to "make another selection in this section."

L-1 Discontinue treatment
Resume treatment when anxiety level diminishes

L-2 Continue the treatment as ordered

L-3 Coach the patient on relaxation relaxation techniques

L-4 Discontinue treatment, request change to hand held nebulizer with albuterol 0.5ml in 2cc NS

L-5 Discontinue treatment, check equipment for malfunction

SECTION M

The low pressure alarm sounds on Kathy's ventilator. To solve this problem, which would you check?

Choose as many as you feel are indicated in this section.

M-1 $FEV_{1sec}/FVC\%$

M-2 ventilator settings

M-3 range of motion

M-4 patency of endotracheal tube

M-5 ventilator circuitry

M-6 chest inspection

M-7 muscle strength test

M-8 breath sounds

M-9 resistance to manual ventilation

M-10 vital capacity

M-11 negative inspiratory force

M-12 corneal reflex

M-13 palpation of neck

M-14 patient sensorium

M-15 cuff pressure manometer

M-16 **When you have completed your selections in this section, then develop M-16**

SECTION N

The physician asks for specifics as to how you would like the order written to accomplish IPPB therapy.

Which would you specify?

Choose only one, unless you are directed to "make another selection in this section."

N-1 IPPB 20 cm H_2O with .5 ml bronkosol/2cc NS Q4 hours

N-2 IPPB 20 cm H_2O with .5 ml isoproternol/2cc NS Q4 hours

N-3 IPPB 20 cm H_2O with 1 ml, 0.5% Albuterol, Q6 hours

N-4 IPPB 20cm H2O with 0.5ml 0.5% Albuterol, Q4 hours

SECTION O

Twenty-four hours later, while beginning your shift in the intensive care unit, you note several significant changes in Kathy's condition. She is noticeably pale, her skin is cool to the touch, peak ventilatory pressure of her ventilator has risen 12 cm H_2O since the last check.

To further evaluate this condition, which would you choose?

Choose as many as you feel are indicated in this section.

O-1 vital signs	temp. is [illegible], pulse 122/min, blood pressure 95/55 mmHg**
O-2 urinalysis	normal**
O-3 blood glucose level	normal**
O-4 obtain STAT chest X-ray	obtained, 40% right pneumothorax, infiltrate RUL**
O-5 basal metabolic rate	not done**
O-6 diagnostic chest percussion	hyperresonant, right hemithorax**
O-7 FEV_{1sec}/FVC %	unable to perform**
O-8 Peak inspiratory flow rate	not done**
O-9 Obtain STAT arterial blood gases	Done, pH 7.30, PCO_2 52 mmHg, PO_2 45 mmHg, HCO_3 25 mEq/l**
O-10 Chest auscultation	Diminished breath sounds right hemithorax**
O-11 tracheal position	shifted to the left**
O-12 partial thromboplastin time	not done**
O-13 aminophylline level	
O-14 chest inspection	
O-15 When you have completed your selections in this section, then develop O-15	

Kathy Pope

Clinical Simulation #4

Answers, Explanations, and Scoring

KATHY POPE

The patient is an asthmatic requiring careful management. The problem involves bronchodilator therapy, an adverse reaction, ventilator commitment, solution of a low pressure alarm problem, and recognition/ solution of tension pneumothorax.

SECTION A

Positive Scoring:

A-1, A-11, A-13, A-15, A-17, A-19, and A-18 Are the standard elements of an initial respiratory evaluation.

A-4 and A-9 Are tools to verify your physical findings. They are evidence on which treatment may be initiated.

A-2, A-3, A-6, and A-14 Are helpful, but peripheral to the evaluation. Hence, the lower scoring. Note the typical ABG values indicative of early ventilatory failure.

A-7 Sputum examination could provide evidence of advanced eosiniphilia if Kirschman's spirals, or casts were present.

Zero Scoring:

A-5 Could possibly be helpful in the patients treatment only if there was a non-related abnormality—not a very strong possibility.

Negative Scoring:

A-8 and A-10 Are beyond the scope of a pulmonary evaluation.

A-16 Hemoglobin abnormality is not in question.

A-12 Is not available as it requires specialized instrumentation.

	Possible	My Score
A-1	+2	
A-2	+1	
A-3	+1	
A-4	+2	
A-5	0	
A-6	+1	
A-7	+1	
A-8	- 2	
A-9	+2	
A-10	- 2	
A-11	+2	
A-12	- 2	
A-13	+2	
A-14	+1	
A-15	+2	
A-16	- 2	
A-17	+2	
A-18	+2	
Total	21	

SECTION F

Positive Scoring:

F-2 Is the preferred choice. The blood gases indicate hypoxemia. The pathology of asthma is bronchoconstriction. This course of action and the patients response to it is crucial in the treatment plan.

F-3 Is an alternative, for which you are partially forgiven as it does include bronchodilation. This choice takes you on an alternate route.

Negative Scoring:

F-1 The blood gases do not warrant mechanical ventilation. The "50-50" rule (PCO_2 > 50 mmHg with PO_2 < 50 mmHg) is not in effect.

F-4 The indication for CPAP (or PEEP) is not present (refractory PaO_2 shunt).

F-5 Is dangerous! Asthmatics are prone to adverse reactions when particulate water is instilled in their airways. It is not indicated as there is no evidence of mucocilicary elevator impairment or need to add water to the airway.

	Possible	My Score
F-1	- 3	
F-2	+ 3	
F-3	+ 1	
F-4	- 3	
F-5	- 3	
Total	+ 3	

ALTERNATE ROUTE
SECTION N

Positive Scoring:

N-3 and N-4 Are the preferrable answers due to the fact Albuterol has the least possibility of Beta 1 side effects. A 0.5% solution contains 5 milligrams/ml.

N-3 Is a heavy dosage as 1 ml would contain 10 mg, understandable given the severity of the asthmatic attack.

N-4 Is the standard dosage of 2.5 mg.

Zero Scoring:

Both N-1 and N-2 Are choices where possible advantages of bronchodilation are offset by the hazards of Beta 1 side effects. In view of the fact a better choice was available, the scoring is zero.

	Possible	My Score
N-1	0	
N-2	0	
N-3	+1	
N-4	+1	
Total	**+1**	

SECTION J

Positive Scoring:

J-3 Is the preferred choice. A venturi mask with a maximum safe dosage of supplemental oxygen is indicated. Prior information describes a hyperventilating patient (PCO_2 32 mmHg, respiratory rate 30/min.) Albuterol is the preferred bronchodilator due to its minimal Beta 1 side effects and duration of action.

J-1 and J-2 Are acceptable, viable options as they meet the criteria for oxygenation and bronchodilation. Isoproternol is potent, short acting, and strongly associated with the Beta 1 response. A nasal cannula is less desireable as the FIO_2 would be diminished by hyperventilation.

Note: The candidate should be aware that ipatropium bromide could have been factored into this asthmatic problem. Be aware of its mode of action and use in the treatment of asthmatics!

Negative Scoring:

J-4 Is inappropriate. Oxygen via a simple mask requires a minimum flow of 4LPM to assure flushing of CO_2 from thc mask.

J-5 Aerosol therapy is an unacceptable risk as is a potential mediator of bronchospasm in the hypersensitive airways of the asthmatic.

	Possible	My Score
J-1	+ 1	
J-2	+ 1	
J-3	+ 3	
J-4	- 3	
J-5	- 3	
Total	+ 3	

ALTERNATE ROUTE
SECTION L

Positive Scoring:

L-4 Is the viable choice. The bridge statement describes an asthmatic with increased, not decreased, bronchospasm. The combination of air flow and particulate water have produced a paradoxical reaction. This is not at all unusual in a patient of this category.

Negative Scoring:

L-1, L-2, and L-3 Are futile. Bronchospasm in the asthmatic is a physiologic response, for which no amount of waiting, coaching, etc. will help.

L-5 The problem does not lie with the equipment. The problem is a paradoxical response on the part of the patient.

	Possible	My Score
L-1	- 3	
L-2	- 3	
L-3	- 3	
L-4	+ 1	
L-5	- 3	
Total	**+ 1**	

SECTION K

Positive Scoring:

K-1 and K-4 Are viable alternatives. Atropine (an anticholinergic) is indicated when a patient cannot tolerate sympathimometics. A reduction to the standard 0.5 ml (2.5 mg) albuterol dosage is also indicated.

Negative Scoring:

K-2 and K-3 Are prophylactic antibiotic asthmatic drugs. They are not indicated to treat the acute attack.

K-5 Is not a viable option.

	Possible	My Score
K-1	+3	
K-2	- 3	
K-3	- 3	
K-4	+3	
K-5	- 3	
Total	+3	

SECTION B

Positive Scoring:

B-4 The bridge statement describes intractable asthma. Kathy will be needing close monitoring in an intensive care situation.

B-8 The blood gases now indicate acute ventilatory failure. She has tired and can no longer sustain oxygenation by hyperventilating.

Prudent and necessary during her course of treatment would be:

B-2 To ward off impending infections

B-3 Standard procedure

B-5 To monitor change of degree of obstruction

B-11 IV aminophylline is toxic beyond a certain level

B-12 X-Rays will be necessary to monitor the infiltrates for progress as therapy gets underway.

Zero Scoring:

B-9 Serum electrolytes are monitored routinely as a precaution when fluid is being infused and fluid balance is in question.

Negative Scoring:

B-1 A blood borne infection is not evident.

B-6 Is not indicated.

B-7 Is premature.

B-10 Is not indicated.

B-13 Would require catheterization, not indicated at this point.

B-14 Right heart failure is not in question.

B-15 There is no evidence that alveolar abnormality is the source of the problem. It is purely an airways disease.

	Possible	My Score
B-1	- 1	
B-2	+ 1	
B-3	+ 1	
B-4	+ 2	
B-5	+ 2	
B-6	- 2	
B-7	- 2	
B-8	+ 2	

	Possible	My Score
B-9	0	
B-10	- 2	
B-11	+ 1	
B-12	+ 2	
B-13	- 2	
B-14	- 2	
B-15	- 2	
Total	**11**	

SECTION E

Positive Scoring:

E-4 The clinical presentation, the course of the illness, and the arterial blood gases mandate commitment to mechanical ventilation. The patient has fatigued to the point where she is no longer able to hyperventilate to maintain an adequate PO_2. She has slipped into acute ventilatory failure. This is typical of a severe attack of asthma.

Negative Scoring:

E-1 and E-2 Have already proven unsuccessful.

E-3 Could possibly improve oxygenation, but it would not address the serious acid-base imbalance.

	Possible	My Score
E-1	- 3	
E-2	- 3	
E-3	- 3	
E-4	+ 3	
Total	+ 3	

SECTION C

Positive Scoring:

C-3 and C-5 Are the preferable, equally scored choices. They are more adaptable to the difficult task of ventilating an asthmatic, who are amongst the most difficult to mechanically ventilate. Higher than normal pressures are required. The patients are extremely uncomfortable/panic stricken. The best technology may not be enough.

C-1 Would be adequate, but a third choice in light of lack of SIMV, low pressure alarms, and pressure support capabilities offered by the options.

Negative Scoring:

C-2 Is not acceptable due to its pressure cycling principle. Also, it is not alarmed suitably to be left unattended.

C-4 is an infant ventilator, exclusively.

	Possible	My Score
C-1	+ 1	
C-2	- 3	
C-3	+ 3	
C-4	- 3	
C-5	+ 3	
Total	+ 3	

SECTION G

Positive Scoring:

G-2 Has the proper tidal volume (12 x 46kg = 500+ml). The patient in status asthmaticus can be expected to be a difficult ventilatory problem for good reason. The flow rate of the gas produces bronchospasm, severe discomfort, and asynchrony. Heavy sedation is the norm rather than the exception. It is a prudent course of action prior to ventilator commitment.

G-1 Is a lesser, but acceptable option as the tidal volume, rate and FIO_2 are all acceptable.

Negative Scoring:

G-3 and G-4 Contain inadequate tidal volumes.

G-5 Contains an excessive tidal volume.

	Possible	My Score
G-1	+ 1	
G-2	+ 3	
G-3	- 3	
G-4	- 3	
G-5	- 3	
Total	+ 3	

ALTERNATE ROUTE
SECTION I

Positive Scoring:

I-4 Now mandates sedation of the patient. In this situation a slower flow rate is preferable to minimize bronchospasm. Note the drop from 30 lpm to 25 lpm.

Negative Scoring:

I-1 Would be counterproductive.

I-2 Could have some beneficial effects pertaining to improvement of distribution of ventilation, but would not have any benefit in combating bronchospasm and "fighting the ventilator."

I-3 Would be of no benefit in solution of this immediate problem.

I-5 Would hyperventilate the patient.

	Possible	My Score
I-1	- 3	
I-2	- 3	
I-3	- 3	
I-4	+ 3	
I-5	- 3	
Total	**+ 3**	

SECTION M

Positive Scoring:

M-2 Would eliminate the possibility of a "knob twister" having changed the setting.

M-5 A leak or disconnect could very well by the culprit.

M-6 Bilateral movement, but diminished, would cause one to suspect escape of inspired gas somewhere.

M-8 Is an indication that gas is escaping around an improperly, inflated endotracheal tube cuff. The gas is gurgling through secretions, above the cuff.

M-13 Would also add to this suspicion.

M-14 Indicates improper ventilation is effecting the patients physiology and sensorium.

M-15 Confirms the suspicion. Gas is escaping around the cuff.

M-9 Also points to a leak in the system.

Negative Scoring:

M-1 A heavily sedated patient is incapable of performing this test.

M-3 Is a physical therapy procedure. .

M-4 Would cause the high pressure alarm to sound-not low pressure.

M-7 Is not relevant.

M-10 Is the same as M-1.

M-11 Would be of no help in the solution of the immediate problem.

M-12 Is the same as M-11.

	Possible	My Score
M-1	- 2	
M-2	+ 1	
M-3	- 2	
M-4	- 2	
M-5	+ 2	
M-6	+ 2	
M-7	- 2	
M-8	+ 2	
M-9	+ 1	
M-10	- 2	
M-11	- 2	
M-12	- 2	
M-13	+ 1	
M-14	+ 1	
M-15	+ 2	
Total	**12**	

SECTION O

Positive Scoring:

O-1 Reveals tachycardia and a precipitously low blood pressure—a result of excessive pressure in the thorax O-6, O-10, O-11 and O-14 all point to pneumothorax.

O-4 Positively confirms your findings.

O-9 Accurately guages the degree of impairment the pneumothorax has caused.

Negative Scoring:

O-2, O-3, O-5, and O-12 Are non-respiratory tests of no value in the solution to this problem.

O-7 and O-8 Are non-viable, effort dependent and irrelevant to the problem.

O-13 Aminophylline levels, when toxic, result in arrythmias-not in question or a part of the problem.

	Possible	My Score
O-1	+ 1	
O-2	- 2	
O-3	- 2	
O-4	+ 2	
O-5	- 2	
O-6	+ 2	
O-7	- 2	
O-8	- 2	
O-9	+ 2	
O-10	+ 1	
O-11	+ 2	
O-12	- 2	
O-13	- 2	
O-14	+ 2	
Total	**12**	

SECTION H

Positive Scoring:

H-3 Is the preferable answer. A chest tube adapts to negative pressure which will be necessary for ongoing positive pressure ventilation.

H-5 Is forgiveable in that it would correct the underlying problem. This solution would be more applicable to an emergency procedure, and, on a patient not undergoing positive pressure ventilation.

Negative Scoring:

H-1 Positive pressure is the cause of the pneumothorax. More positive pressure would be counterproductive.

H-2 The clinical signs and X-Ray data denote pneumothorax to be the underlying cause of the problem. It is not right mainstem intubation.

H-4 Is indicated where all ACLS measures have failed and the mechanical ventilation maneuvers (super PEEP, 100% oxygen) have proven inadequate to sustain oxygenation.

	Possible	My Score
H-1	- 3	
H-2	- 3	
H-3	+ 3	
H-4	- 3	
H-5	+ 1	
Total	+ 3	

KATHY POPE

ROUTE AND SCORING

Route	Possible	My Score
A	21	
F	3	
N	[1]	
J	3	
L	[1]	
K	3	
B	11	
E	3	
C	3	
G	3	
I	[3]	
M	12	
O	12	
H	3	
Total	**77**	

Optimal route passing score <u>52</u>
All alternate routes <u>53</u>

KATHY POPE

REFERENCES

1. Burton, Hodgkins: **Respiratory Care a Guide to Clinical Practice, 2nd Edition,** Lippincott, 1984. (Pages 266, 438, 456-498, 556-576, 648, 651, 940-945)

2. Mitchell & Petty: **Synopsis of Clinical Pulmonary Disease, 3rd Edition,** C.V. Mosby, 1982. (Page 51)

3. Pilbeam: **Mechanical Ventilation Physiologic Applications and Clinical Applications,** Multi-Media Publishing, Inc., C.V. Mosby, 1986. (Pages 53-60, 103-109, 163-205, 172-174, 273-296)

4. Shapiro: **Clinical Application of Respiratory Care, 3rd Edition,** Year Book Medical Publishers, 1985. (Pages 62-68, 76-79, 379-407)

Irma Torres

Clinical Simulation #5

Problem

IRMA TORRES

You are a staff therapist in a 320-bed community hospital. Your pager sounds to report to the emergency room. There, the charge nurse requests your assistance with Irma Torres. She is 68 years old, her chief complaint is shortness of breath, and general malaise. She has a tracheostomy scar and a past medical history of recurring respiratory infections.

NOW GO TO SECTION A

SECTION A

Which of the following would you include in your initial assessment?

Choose as many as you feel are indicated in this section.

A-1 Temperature	38.3 C, 100.9 F**
A-2 Breath sounds	Decreased in both bases**
A-3 Range of motion of extremeties	
A-4 Level of consciousness	Alert and oriented**
A-5 Respiratory rate and pattern	30/min. labored, Intercostal retractions**
A-6 Posture	Semi Fowler's**
A-7 Pulse and blood pressure	110/min. 165/105 mmHg**
A-8 Urine output	
A-9 Skin color	No cyanosis noted**
A-10 Capillary refill	Normal**
A-11 Babinski reflex	
A-12 Tracheal position	Midline**
A-13 Response to pain	
A-14 Bowel sounds	
A-15 Pedal edema	Absent**
A-16 Sputum production	4 Ounces over the past 12 hours**
A-17 Thoracic symmetry	Equal bilateral movement**
A-18 Diagnostic chest percussion	Diminished, dull, right and left lower lobes**
A-19 **When you have completed your selections in this section, develop A-19**	Go to Section K**

SECTION B

While checking another ventilator in the intensive care unit, you hear the high pressure alarm of Mrs. Torres' ventilator sounding. To determine the cause, which would you evaluate?

Choose as many as you feel are indicated in this section.

B-1 Check the ventilator's power source	
B-2 Auscultate the patient's chest	Diminished sounds, right hemithorax**
B-3 Check ventilator controls	Unchanged**
B-4 Check endotracheal tube for patency	Patent**
B-5 Increase the high pressure alarm control setting 10 cm H_2O	
B-6 Check circuitry connections	
B-7 Obtain lateral decubitus, chest x-ray	
B-8 Perform diagnostic chest percussion	Marked dullness, right hemithorax**
B-9 Disconnect patient, manually ventilate	Increased resistance to ventilation**
B-10 Check position of the trachea	Shifted slightly to the right**
B-11 Perform estimated shunt study (Q_s/Q_t)	
B-12 Recommend bronchogram	
B-13 **When you have completed your selections in this section, then develop B-13**	Go to Section F**

SECTION C

Which would you recommend now?

Choose only one, unless you are directed to "make another selection in this section."

C-1 Administer 20% acetylcysteine directly into the endotracheal tube

C-2 Perform fiberoptic bronchoscopy

C-3 Replace on ventilator, increase TV to 1000 ml, utilize inspiratory plateau

C-4 Perform postural drainage, percussion and vibration

SECTION D

Of the following, which would you recommend next?

Choose only one, unless you are directed to "make another selection in this section."

D-1 Obtain laboratory data and perform diagnostic procedures	Physician agrees; go to section H**
D-2 Administer postural drainage	
D-3 Refer the patient to the hospital's rehabilitation program	
D-4 Intubate the patient	
D-5 Administer IPPB therapy with racemic epinephrine	

SECTION E

The physician asks your recommendations. Which of the following would you suggest?

Choose only one, unless you are directed to "make another selection in this section."

E-1 Intubate, administer CPAP 5 cm H_2O, FIO_2 0.7	Physician disagrees; make another selection in this section.**
E-2 Intubate, administer O_2 via T piece (Briggs adapter) FIO_2 0.7	Physician disagrees; make another selection in this section.**
E-3 Intubate and mechanically ventilate	Done; she is transferred to intensive care unit. Go to Section G**
E-4 Intubate, support ventilation via resuscitation bag FIO_2 1.0	Done; she is transferred to intensive care unit. Go to Section [illegible]
E-5 Hyperinflation therapy (IPPB) with 10% acetylcysteine	Physician disagrees; make another selection in this section.**

SECTION F

While manually ventilating the patient, you note Mrs. Torres' blood pressure dropping. It reads 115/60 mmHg. What would you recommend now?

Choose only one, unless you are directed to "make another selection in this section."

F-1	Obtain a chest x-ray stat.	Endotracheal tube properly placed. Collapse of right middle and lower lobes, go to Section C**
F-2	Retract the endotracheal tube 2-3 cm	Done, problem persists**
F-3	Insertion of a chest tube	Physician disagrees, make another selection in this section.**
F-4	Tracheostomy	Physician disagrees, make another selection in this section.**
F-5	Instill 3 cc normal saline, suction the patient	Done, secretions thick and difficult to remove. Problem persists, make another selection in this section.**

SECTION G

The physician asks for your recommendations on ventilator parameters. Mrs. Torres weighs 130 lbs (59 kg).

Choose only one, unless you are directed to "make another selection in this section."

G-1 Assist/Control, FIO_2 0.70, Rate 8, TV 800 ml	Physician agrees, go to Section B**
G-2 IMV Mandatory rate 8, TV 800 ml, FIO_2 0.70	Physician agrees, go to Section B**
G-3 IMV Mandatory rate 8, TV 800 ml, PEEP 10 cm H_2O, FIO_2 0.30	Physician disagrees, make another selection in this section.**
G-4 CPAP mode, PEEP 10 cm H_2O, FIO_2 0.70	Physician disagrees, make another selection in this section.**
G-5 Control mode, rate 10, TV 700 ml, FIO_2 0.70	Physician agrees, go to Section B**
G-6 Control mode, rate 16, TV 500 ml, FIO_2 0.40	Physician disagrees, make another selection in this section.**
G-7 Control mode, rate 10, PEEP 10 cm H_2O, FIO_2 0.30	Physician disagrees, make another selection in this section.**

SECTION H

Mrs. Torres is admitted to the hospital's pulmonary service. Which of the following would you recommend?

Choose as many as you feel are indicated in this section.

H-1 Cardiac enzymes	
H-2 Chest x-ray	Consolidation of l Narrowed trachea midpoint of trach
H-3 Urine pH	
H-4 Measured P50	
H-5 Gram stain of sputum	Numerous coloni
H-6 Sputum culture and sensitivity	Ordered**
H-7 Lactate level	
H-8 Measured % shunt (Q_s/Q_t)	
H-9 Prothrombin clotting time	
H-10 12 Lead ECG	Normal sinus rhy
H-11 % Of deadspace (V_d/V_t)	
H-12 Arterial blood gases	pH 7.45 PCO_2 35 mmHg, HCO_3 24
H-13 Lung scan	Noted**
H-14 Flow volume loop study	
H-15 CBC	Hb 13.5 grams %, WBC 10,000 mm^3
H-16 Determination of FRC	
H-17 Pulmonary compliance	
H-18 Pulmonary angiogram	
H-19 Serum electrolytes	Within normal li
H-20 **When you have completed your selections in this section, then develop H-20**	Go to Section I.**

SECTION I

Which of the following would be your next recommendation?

Choose only one, unless you are directed to "make another selection in this section."

I-1 Maintain present therapy, monitor

I-2 Intubate and mechanically ventilate

I-3 Intubate and support ventilation via resuscitation bag FIO_2 0.70

I-4 Administer 0_2 via partial rebreather mask
Obtain arterial blood gas.

I-5 Administer hyperinflation therapy (IPPB) with racemic epinephrine

SECTION J

Mrs. Torres becomes unresponsive. Pulse is 140/min., blood pressure 170/115. Manual ventilation is difficult. What would you recommend now?

Choose only one, unless you are directed to "make another selection in this section."

J-1 Mechanically ventilate

J-2 Perform ventilation/perfusion scan

J-3 Continue present therapy, monitor

J-4 Administer hyperinflation therapy (IPPB) FIO_2 1.0

J-5 Administer O_2 via partial rebreather mask

SECTION K

The emergency room physician asks for your recommendations initiate therapy. Which would you suggest?

Choose only one, unless you are directed to "make another selection in this section."

K-1 Bronchodilator therapy
Albuterol 2.5 mg

K-2 Aerosol therapy via ultrasonic
nebulizer

K-3 Obtain arterial blood gases

K-4 Institute oxygen therapy via
nasal cannula 4 L/min.

Done; go to Section D**

K-5 Administer IPPB therapy with
5 mg isoetherine

SECTION L

One hour later, you are paged by the pulmonary charge nurse. She informs you, Mrs. Torres has become extremely short of breath. Proceeding to her room immediately, you note the patient is cyanotic and disoriented. What would you do at this point?

Choose only one, unless you are directed to "make another selection in this section."

L-1 Continue present therapy, monitor the patient	
L-2 Administer O_2 via partial rebreathing mask. Obtain an ABG in 15 minutes.	Done, pH 7.20, PaO_2 68 mmHg, PCO_2 48 mmHg, HCO_3 23 mEq/L go to Section F**
L-3 Obtain a STAT ABG	
L-4 Intubate and ventilate	
L-5 Institute postural drainage, percussion, and vibration Q2 hrs.	

SECTION M

What would you recommend now?

Choose only one, unless you are directed to "make another selection in this section."

M-1 Refer the patient to the hospital's rehabilitation program

M-2 Administer oxygen via nasal cannula 4 L/min.

M-3 Administer oxygen via 35% venturi mask

M-4 Intubate the patient

M-5 Administer postural drainage, percussion, and vibration

M-6 Monitor the patient, no therapy is needed at this time

Irma Torres

Clinical Simulation #5

Answers,
Explanations,
and Scoring

IRMA TORRES

This problem involves management of a compromised patient with respiratory complications. You are required to manage her sudden deterioration and subsequent ventilator and mucus plugging problems.

SECTION A

Positive Scoring:

A preliminary patient assessment would include: inspection (A-1, A-4, A-5, A-6, A-7, A-9, A-12, A-15, A-17, and A-18), percussion (A-18), and auscultation (A-2). An emergency room patient is routinely monitored for temperature, pulse, and respiratory rate—all readily available at the bedside and of importance to the assessment of the patient.

Skin color (A-9) and capillary refill (A-10) are general indications of cardiac output. Pedal edema (A-15) and sputum production (A-16) would be indicators of underlying cardiac on respiratory disease.

Negative Scoring:

Range of motion (A-3) is extraneous to a pulmonary assessment (A-8) urine output is information not available until hospital admission. (A-11) is extraneous to a pulmonary assessment. Babinski reflex is a neurological sign. It, also, has no place in a respiratory workup. Response to pain (A-13) is not only unwarranted—it would be cruel. Bowel sounds (A-14) again, outside the scope of a respiratory assessment.

	Possible	My Score
A-1	+2	+2
A-2	+3	+3
A-3	- 3	
A-4	+1	+1
A-5	+3	+3
A-6	+1	+1
A-7	+1	+1
A-8	- 3	
A-9	+1	+1
A-10	+1	+1
A-11	- 2	
A-12	+1	0
A-13	- 3	
A-14	- 3	
A-15	+3	+3
A-16	+1	+1
A-17	+1	+1
A-18	+3	+3
Total	22	21

SECTION K

Positive Scoring:

K-4 Proper action, initially is action to relieve the patient's respiratory distress. All signs and symptoms indicate hypoxemia. The "first" therapy to institute supplemental oxygen.

K-3 If you chose to draw an arterial blood gas, you were directed to an alternate route. An ABG would define the degree of hypoxemia and would be central to later therapeutic measures, but not the first course of action. It merits a lesser possible score for that reason.

Negative Scoring:

Bronchodilator therapy (K-1 and K-5) are not indicated at this juncture. Quite possibly, it might be later in the course of treatment. However, a patient eliciting dyspnea, fever, and lung consolidation suggests the major, underlying cause to be infection—not bronchoconstriction.

Aerosol therapy (K-2) is not indicated. Their is no evidence of dried, insippated secretions or the need to add water to the airways.

	Possible	My Score
K-1	- 3	
K-2	- 3	
K-3	+ 1	
K-4	+ 3	+3
K-5	- 3	
Total	**+ 3**	+3

SECTION M
(ALTERNATE ROUTE)

Positive Scoring:

M-2 and M-3 If you chose this route, you are now forced back to the main route. The arterial blood gases mandate supplemental oxygen therapy. It is immaterial which delivery appliance you chose.

Negative Scoring:

M-1 and M-6 Are obviously non-contributory to the solution of the immediate problem. Intubation (M-4) would be premature and perhaps, totally unnecessary prior to assessing the effect of conservative oxygen therapy.

	Possible	My Score
M-1	- 3	
M-2	+ 3	
M-3	+ 3	
M-4	- 3	
M-5	- 3	
M-6	- 3	

SECTION D

Positive Scoring:

D-1 Before the patient can be managed properly, more information must be gathered. Such basic tests, such as X-rays, ABG, and microscopic sputum examination will define a precise course of treatment.

Negative Scoring:

Note the similarity between this decision making section and a multiple choice question. By using the information you have gathered and the scenario as the body of the question, which is the "one best response". (D-3) and (D-4) are obviously wrong. Postural drainage, percussion, and vibration (D-2) might be indicated, but as yet, we have no hard evidence of atelectasis or retained secretions. IPPB with racemic epinephrine (D-5) may be eliminated for the same reason, plus, there is no indication for administration of a decongestant, alpha adrenergic drug.

Note: Our patient is still in the emergency room, in early ventilatory failure, awaiting further treatment.

	Possible	My Score
D-1	+ 3	+3
D-2	- 3	
D-3	- 3	
D-4	- 3	
D-5	- 3	
Total	**+ 3**	+3

SECTION H

Positive Scoring:

H-2, H-5, H-6, and H-12 Central to the treatment of the patient is information which locates the infection, defines a fixed airway obstruction, denotes the infecting organism, and will guide the physician for specific antibiotic therapy. The ABG also rules out chronic lung disease. Most likely, Mrs. Torres' recurring respiratory infections are a result of tracheal stenosis secondary to tracheostomy during a previous hospitalization.

H-14 and H-15 Peripheral information which will contribute to her course of treatment is a flow volume loop study to determine the extent of the tracheal stenosis, a CBC to determine the condition of the O_2 transport mechanism, as well as the extent of her gram (+) cocci lung infection.

Zero Scoring:

H-10 A 12 lead ECG is not harmful, but also not indicated at this time.

Negative Scoring:

Mrs. Torres is still in the emergency room unintubated. This makes shunt studies(H-8), lung scan(H-13), determination of compliance(H-17), FRC(H-16) and % of deadspace(H-11), if not impossible, extremely difficult and time consuming.

H-1 Cardiac enzymes are not indicated. Urine pH(H-3), P50(H-4), lactate levels(H-7), prothrombin clotting time(H-9), pulmonary angiogram(H-18) and serum electrolytes(H-19) would be costly, time consuming, and non-contributing to an effective regimen of treatment.

	Possible	My Score
H-1	- 2	
H-2	+ 3	+3
H-3	- 1	
H-4	- 2	
H-5	+ 2	+2
H-6	+ 2	+2
H-7	- 1	
H-8	- 3	
H-9	- 2	
H-10	0	0
H-11	- 3	
H-12	+ 3	+3
H-13	- 2	-2
H-14	+ 1	•
H-15	+ 1	+1
H-16	- 2	
H-17	- 2	
H-18	- 2	
H-19	- 1	-1
Total	**12**	8

SECTION L

Positive Scoring:

L-2 Mrs. Torres' condition is precipitous. If not treated immediately, her life could be in danger. Cyanosis indicates a rapid deterioration of her condition and a serious depletion of blood oxygen stores. Proper action is to increase the present FIO_2 (34%) to 60-90%. After accomplishing this, an arterial blood gas is indicated to assess results. The blood gas results (15 minutes later) denotes conversion of early ventilatory failure to acute respiratory failure.

If you chose L-3 (arterial blood gases immediately) the penalty is loss of two (2) possible points and direction through an alternate route.

Negative Scoring:

L-1 and L-5 are obviously wrong as they do not address the immediate, central problem of acute ventilatory failure. (L-4) At this point, it would be premature to intubate and mechanically ventilate. The patient may respond, favorably, to an increased increment of FIO_2.

	Possible	My Score
L-1	- 3	
L-2	+ 3	+3
L-3	+ 1	
L-4	- 3	
L-5	- 3	
Total	+ 3	+3

SECTION I
(ALTERNATE ROUTE)

Positive Scoring:

I-2 In this section you may get back to the main route by instituting mechanical ventilation. You may also continue along an alternate route by electing to ventilate via a resuscitation bag (I-3). The latter merely postpones the inevitable.

Negative Scoring:

I-1 Maintenance of present therapy would be severly detrimental to patients health.

I-4 If you chose to institute a higher FIO_2 utilizing a partial rebreather mask, you are forced to retreat to Section E where mechanical ventilation may commence. This will allow you to recoup some, but not all, points.

I-5 Selection of this option is inappropriate for this situation.

	Possible	My Score
I-1	- 3	
I-2	+ 3	
I-3	+ 1	
I-4	0	
I-5	- 3	
Total	**+ 3**	

SECTION E

Positive Scoring:

E-3 The indications are present for ventilator commitment (the 50-50 rule).

E-4 Leads you to an alternate route. The penalty is two (2) possible points — This choice, although not the best course of action, is forgiveable.

Negative Scoring:

E-1 and E-2 Require spontaneous breathing, which has proven inadequate. (E-5) IPPB would be temporary in nature. 10% Acetylcysteine, a mucolytic, from the information now at hand, may or may not be indicated.

	Possible	My Score
E-1	- 3	
E-2	- 3	
E-3	+ 3	+3
E-4	+ 1	
E-5	- 3	
Total	+ 3	+3

SECTION J
(ALTERNATE ROUTE)

Positive Scoring:

You are on an alternate route. In this section you are forced back onto the main route.

J-1 The most appropriate selection for this patient who is rapidly deteriorating.

J-5 Prolongs the inevitable intubation of this patient.

Negative Scoring:

All other options are obviously wrong!

	Possible	My Score
J-1	+ 3	
J-2	- 1	
J-3	- 1	
J-4	- 1	
J-5	+ 2	
Total	**+ 3**	

SECTION G

Positive Scoring:

G-1 and G-2 The initial tidal volume is calculated at the accepted 12-15 ml/kg.—800 ml is within that range. A rate of 8 computes to (8 x 800 ml) a minute volume (V_e) of 6.4 liters. A high FIO_2 would be indicated, initially, prior to titrating an acceptable P_aO_2. The control mode (G-5) meets the criteria but awards less points as the patient is breathing spontaneously. Control is not specifically indicated, but is forgiveable.

Negative Scoring:

G-3, G-6, and G-7 Could be eliminated at the outset due to their unsatisfactory (low) FIO_2.

CPAP requires spontaneous breathing. Its inadequacy is documented by the previous arterial blood gas.

PEEP, also, would eliminate G-4 and G-7. Shunt has not been established as a cause of hypoxia/ hypoxemia. Contrary to popular usage, PEEP is indicated only, in the treatment of physiologic shunt (refractory P_aO_2).

	Possible	My Score
G-1	+3	
G-2	+3	
G-3	- 3	
G-4	- 3	
G-5	+2	+2
G-6	- 3	
G-7	- 3	
Total	+3	+2

SECTION B

This section tests your troubleshooting skills—given—the ventilator's high pressure alarm is sounding.

Positive Scoring:

B-2 Pneumothorax, bronchospasm, or excessive secretions would be recognizable on auscultation. All could cause the high pressure alarm to sound.

B-3 Yes. Unauthorized changes of flow, volume, or rate could cause the alarm to sound.

B-4 Dried secretions or kinking of the ET tube could be the cause of excessive pressure.

B-8 Chest percussion is diagnostic of pneumothorax, and for consolidation—both possible causes.

B-9 Yes. Manual ventilation would define a patient vs. machine problem.

B-10 A tracheal shift would be indicative of pneumothorax or severe atelectasis.

Negative Scoring:

B-1 Ventilator disconnect alarms are designed to be loud and unique. They are impossible not to recognize.

B-5 No. The alarm would not sound, but the problem persists.

B-6 No. A low pressure alarm would sound—not high pressure.

B-7 A lateral decubitus x-ray would be time consuming and of doubtful value.

B-11 The means (Swan-Ganz catheter) are unavailable—also, of questionable value.

B-12 Not indicated for correction of the problem.

	Possible	My Score
B-1	- 1	
B-2	+ 2	+2
B-3	+ 2	+2
B-4	+ 3	+3
B-5	- 3	
B-6	- 2	
B-7	- 3	
B-8	+ 3	+3
B-9	+ 3	+3
B-10	+ 2	+2
B-11	- 1	
B-12	- 3	
Total	**14**	15

SECTION F

Positive Scoring:

F-1 Central to the resolution of the problem is determination of the cause of Mrs. Torres' deterioration. As all other causes are ruled out in the troubleshooting section (B), an x-ray is the only recourse to ascertain the loss of lung volume. The results tell you air is being denied entry to the right middle and lower lobes.

The drop in blood pressure is a secondary indicator the patient is in a precipitous crisis.

Zero Scoring:

F-5 If you chose to suction the patient, you are not penalized. This action holds some promise of alleviating the problem, but holds no guarantees. More aggressive therapy (therapeutic bronchoscopy) is available for you to utilize.

Negative Scoring:

From the information provided, there is no evidence of pneumothorax (F-3), or that the endotracheal tube is in the right mainstem bronchus (F-2). Auscultation, diagnostic percussion, and a tracheal right shift all indicate massive consolidation of the right lung fields. (F-4) Not indicated at this time.

	Possible	My Score
F-1	+ 3	+3
F-2	- 3	−3
F-3	- 3	
F-4	- 3	
F-5	0	
Total	+ 3	0

SECTION C

Positive Scoring:

C-2 Fiberoptic bronchoscopy is the preferable choice. This procedure allows visualization to the ninth generation bronchi, and also has the ability to selectively suction, if necessary.

C-1 and C-3 Are alternatives with some promise of success, but with not guarantees. The fact that we have a deteriorating patient with two collapsed lobes mandate immediate, aggressive therapy.

Negative Scoring:

C-4 Although an indication for the treatment and prophylaxis of atelectasis is inappropriate in the face of a medical emergency.

	Possible	My Score
C-1	+ 1	
C-2	+ 3	
C-3	+ 1	
C-4	- 3	-3
Total	+ 3	-3

IRMA TORRES

Route	Possible	My Score
A	22	21
↓ K	3	3
↓ D ↘ M	3 / 3	3
↓ H	12	8
↓ L	3	3
↘ I	3	
↓ E	3	3
↘ J	3	
↓ G	3	+2
↓ B	14	15
↓ F	3	0
↓ C	3	-3
Total	**69**	55

Optimal Route Passing Score **47**
Alternate Route IJE Passing Score **48**

IRMA TORRES

REFERENCES

1. Burton, Hodgkins: **Respiratory Care a Guide to Clinical Practice, 2nd Edition,** Lippincott, 1984. (Pages 282-297, 438, 796)

2. Pilbeam: **Mechanical Ventilation Physiologic Applications and Clinical Applications,** Multi-Media Publishing, Inc., C.V. Mosby, 1986. (Pages 44-46)

3. Shapiro: **Clinical Application of Respiratory Care, 3rd Edition,** Year Book Medical Publishers, 1985. (Pages 62-68, 176-187, 379-407)

Jim Burgey

Clinical Simulation #6

Problem

JIM BURGEY

You are a night shift respiratory therapist in a 250-bed community hospital. You are paged to the emergency room to assist in the care of a patient. Jim Burgey, the victim of a one car accident, has suffered severe trauma to the head and face. The emergency room charge nurse requests your help in the ventilatory management of the patient pending the arrival of the on-call emergency physician. Mr. Burgey is approximately 6 feet tall and weighs 185 lbs. (84 kg).

NOW GO TO SECTION A

SECTION A

Which of the following would you choose to assess the patient?

Choose as many as you feel are indicated in this section.

A-1 Pulmonary artery pressure	
A-2 Tidal volume	Unable to measure due to facial laceration**
A-3 Cardiac output	
A-4 Minute volume	Unable to assess due to facial laceration**
A-5 Respiratory rate and pattern	Difficult to assess, pattern is ataxic**
A-6 Urine output	
A-7 Level of Conscious	Non-responsive, non-specific, random movement**
A-8 Skin color	Pale**
A-9 Vital capacity	
A-10 Pupillary response	Present, but unequal**
A-11 Chest wall movement	Equal bilaterally, irregular**
A-12 Central venous pressure	
A-13 Gag reflex	
A-14 Pedal edema	Absent**
A-15 Evidence of thoracic trauma (bruises)	None**
A-16 Evidence of long bone fractures	None**
A-17 Blood pressure and pulse	90/60 mmHg, 115/min.**
A-18 Intraocular pressure	
A-19 **When you have completed your selections in this section, then develop A-19**	Go to Section F**

SECTION B

24 Hours later, ABG's are pH 7.48, PCO_2 32 mmHg PO_2 68 mmHg, HCO_3^- 24.5 mEq/l. Intercranial pressure is 4 mmHg. Chest x-rays denote bilateral areas of patchy infiltrates. The patients static compliance is .023 L/cm H_2O — on a downward trend.

What changes would you recommend?

Choose only one, unless you are directed to "make another selection in this section."

B-1 Add 5 cm H_2O PEEP, FIO_2 0.40

Physician agrees, go to Section F**

B-2 Maintain present parameters, monitor patient

B-3 Increase FIO_2 to 0.8

B-4 Add 5 cm H_2O PEEP, FIO_2 0.50, increase tidal volume 150 ml

B-5 Increase flow rate 5 L/min.

B-6 Increase respiratory rate to 14/min.

SECTION C

What would you recommend now?

Choose only one, unless you are directed to "make another selection in this section."

C-1 Intubate, Ventilate via resuscitation bag, FIO_2 1.0	Physician agrees, go to Section K**
C-2 Maintain present therapy, monitor patient	Physician disagrees, make another selection in this section.**
C-3 Hyperinflation therapy, FIO_2 1.0	Physician disagrees, make another selection in this section.**
C-4 Increase FIO_2 to 0.8	Physician disagrees, make another selection in this section.**
C-5 Administer Albuterol, 3 mg. via hand-held nebulizer	Physician disagrees, make another selection in this section.**

SECTION D

Which of the following procedures/data would you suggest?

Choose as many as you feel are indicated in this section.

D-1 Urinalysis	
D-2 Chest x-ray	Lung field clear. No vertebral or rib fractures**
D-3 Arterial blood gases	FIO_2 0.40, pH 7.25, PCO_2 53 mmHg, PO_2 48 mmHg, HCO_3 23 mEq/l**
D-4 Blood glucose	
D-5 Lung scan	
D-6 Head and neck x-rays	Skull fractures. Evidence of cerebral contusion. Cervical vertebrae intact.**
D-7 Serum electrolytes	Normal**
D-8 Sputum culture	
D-9 Cardiac enzymes	
D-10 Complete blood count (CBC) and differential	Not done**
D-11 Hematocrit/Hemoglobin	
D-12 P-50	
D-13 Negative inspiratory Force (NIF)	
D-14 ECG monitor	Sinus tachycardia rate 120/min.**
D-15 When you have completed your selections in this section, then develop D-15	Go to Section C**

SECTION E

Working your shift the next night, data on Mr. Burgey is as follows:

VD/VT 42%
% Shunt 45%
Compliance .028 l/cm H_2O
Intercranial pressure — discontinued
$P(A\text{-}a)_{02}$ (on 100% O_2) 360 mmHg
X-ray report: Resolving infiltrates compared to previous film

FIO_2 0.40
PEEP 10 cm H_2O
ABG's pH 7.46, PCO_2 36 mmHg, PO_2 84 mmHg, HCO_3, 26 mEq/l
d Turbocurarine — discontinued

What would you recommend now?

Choose only one unless you are directed to "make another selection in this section."

E-1 Maintain present ventilator parameters

Physician agrees, end of problem**

E-2 Increase PEEP to 20 cm H_2O

E-3 Commence weaning procedures

E-4 Increase FIO_2 to 0.50

E-5 Decrease PEEP to 5 cm H_2O

SECTION F

The emergency room physician has not yet arrived. The emergency room charge nurse asks is anything should be done immediately?

What would you recommend?

Choose only one, unless you are directed to "make another selection in this section."

F-1 Obtain laboratory data	
F-2 Intubate and ventilate	
F-3 Administer oxygen via simple mask	
F-4 Administer oxygen via nasal connula	
F-5 Administer oxygen via 40% venturi mask	Done, go to Section [illegible]**

SECTION G

Thirty minutes later, Mr. Burgey's arterial blood gases are: pH 7.36, PCO_2 48 mmHg, PO_2 120 mmHg HCO_3^- 22 mEq/l. The intercranial pressure monitor is reading 12 mmHg.

Which would you suggest now?

Choose only one, unless you are directed to "make another selection in this section."

G-1 Maintain present ventilator parameter

G-2 Control mode, FIO_2 0.40, rate 13, TV 1200 ml

G-3 Control mode, FIO_2 0.30, rate 11, tidal volume 1050 ml

G-4 IMV mode, FIO_2 0.40, rate 10 tidal volume 750 ml, PEEP 5 cm H_2O

G-5 Assist control mode, FIO_2 0.40 machine rate 6, tidal volume 1000 ml, PEEP 5 cm H_2O

SECTION H

One half hour later the patient is restless and "fighting" the ventilator. Spontaneous breaths are approximately 34/min. and continue in an irregular ataxic pattern. Arterial blood gases are: pH 7.31, PCO_2 52 mmHg, PO_2 47 mmHg, HCO_3^- 26 mEq/l.

What would you recommend?

Choose only one, unless you are directed to "make another selection in this section."

H-1 Control mode, FIO_2 0.50, rate 10, tidal volume 1000 ml, Administer d Turbocurarine

Physician agrees, go to section [illegible]

H-2 Maintain present parameters, monitor

H-3 IMV mode, FIO_2 0.80, rate 12, tidal volume 1100 ml

Physician disagrees, make another selection in this section.

H-4 CPAP mode 10 cm H_2O, FIO_2 0.8

H-5 Assist control mode, FIO_2 1.0, rate 14, tidal volume 1100 ml

Physician disagrees, make another selection in this section.

SECTION J

The on-call physician arrives and asks for your recommendations. Meanwhile the non-respiratory aspects of Mr. Burgey's injuries are attended to.

Of the following, which would you choose?

Choose only one, unless you are directed to "make another selection in this section."

J-1 Obtain laboratory data and further evaluate	Physician agrees, go to Section D**
J-2 Intubate and ventilate, FIO_2 1.0	
J-3 Determine the patient's age and past medical history	
J-4 Determine time elapsed from accident to arrival	
J-5 Administer hyperinflation therapy, FIO_2 0.1	

SECTION K

The patient is transferred to the intensive care unit for ongoing treatment. Mechanical ventilation is instituted.

Which would you recommend?

Choose only one, unless you are directed to "make another selection in this section."

K-1 IMV mode, FIO_2 0.5, rate 12, TV 900 ml	Physician agrees, go to Section [illegible]
K-2 Control mode, FIO_2 0.5 rate 10, TV 1000 ml, Administer d Turbocurarine	
K-3 Assist/control, FIO_2 0.5	
K-4 IMV mode, FIO_2 0.5, machine rate 8, TV 1000 ml	
K-5 CPAP mode, 5 cm H_2O, FIO_2 0.8	

Jim Burgey

Clinical Simulation #6

Answers,
Explanations,
and Scoring

JIM BURGEY

This problem requires management of a head trauma patient, initial oxygen therapy, to eventual weaning from a ventilator. Coincidentally, you must have knowledge of control of intercranial pressure via low P_aCO_2.

SECTION A

Mr. Burgey's description depicts a patient with immediate, ventilatory and respiratory problems. He is at risk to ARDS, shock, impaired control of breathing, and elevated intracranial pressure.

Positive Scoring:

A-2, A-4, and A-5 Although unable to assess would be important factors to consider in the care of the patient.

A-7 Is pivotal to the ventilatory management of the patient.

A-8 Easily accomplished and establishes diminished cardiac output, probable hypoxemia and shock.

A-10 Establishes injury to the breathing control centers of the lower brain and/or elevated ICP.

A-11 Determines the absence of flail chest — a distinct possibility and a factor to consider.

A-15 Lung contusion, although absent, could be a central factor.

A-16 Could be a source of fat, pulmonary emboli.

A-17 This, also, establishes the presence of hypoxemia and shock.

Zero Scoring:

A-14 Would be evidence of pre-existing pulmonary disease. Observing the fact would neither harm nor help the patient.

Negative Scoring:

A-1, A-3, A-6, and A-12 Would require instrumentation and cannulation — not in place.

A-13 and A-18 Are outside the scope of a respiratory assessment.

A-9 Obviously unavailable on an unconscious patient.

	Possible	My Score
A-1	- 2	
A-2	+ 2	+2
A-3	- 2	
A-4	+ 2	
A-5	+ 2	+2
A-6	- 2	
A-7	+ 2	+2
A-8	+ 1	+1
A-9	- 2	
A-10	+ 1	+1

	Possible	My Score
A-11	+ 2	+2
A-12	- 2	
A-13	- 2	
A-14	0	0
A-15	+ 2	+2
A-16	+ 2	+2
A-17	+ 1	+1
A-18	- 2	
Total	**17**	15

SECTION F

Positive Scoring:

F-5 Hypoxemia/hypoxia, to an unknown degree has been determined by the initial assessment. Oxygen therapy is indicated. A high flow delivery appliance is required due to the erratic breathing pattern of the patient.

Negative Scoring:

F-1 Obtaining data is essential to accurately and properly treat the patient. However, the first thing to accomplish is addressing the problem of hypoxia/hypoxemia — commence oxygen therapy.

F-2 Intubation and ventilation are distinct possibilities. However no evidence is present for their indications. Oxygen therapy might obviate its need.

F-3 and F-4 Are low flow oxygen delivery systems — inappropriate for an ataxic patient.

	Possible	My Score
F-1	- 1	
F-2	- 3	
F-3	- 2	
F-4	- 3	
F-5	+3	+3
Total	+3	+3

SECTION J

Positive Scoring:

J-1 More data is needed before more specific treatment can be initiated. The most pressing need is to determine the severity of Mr. Burgey's hypoxia/hypoxema and his ability to ventilate.

Negative Scoring:

J-2 Although this option is a distinct possibility, it is still undetermined if the indications exist.

J-3 and J-4 Are of doubtful value to the resolution of the patient's condition. Both choices would waste valuable time.

J-5 Inappropriate under any circumstances. No indications exist for its application.

	Possible	My Score
J-1	+3	+3
J-2	- 3	
J-3	- 3	
J-4	- 3	
J-5	- 3	
Total	+3	+3

SECTION D

Positive Scoring:

D-2 Rib fractures, if present, could have bearing on the respiratory management of the patient.

D-3 Determination of arterial blood gas values are central to the immediate and longer term management of the patient.

D-6 Is helpful as it would have a bearing on the care and handling of the patient— as a "rule out" procedure.

D-11 Hematocrit and Hemoglobin would yield sufficient information to determine the extent of blood loss. Blood loss would relate to oxygen carrying capability.

D-14 An ECG monitor is mildly contributory and a prudent procedure standard in most emergency trauma rooms.

Zero Scoring:

D-9 Not indicated in this situation.

D-10 Is non-contributory.

Negative Scoring:

D-1, D-4, and D-12 Are all beyond the scope of appropriate respiratory or medical care of a head and facial trauma victim.

D-7 Is inappropriate and (D-5) would require moving the patient.

D-8 Also inappropriate. Infection is not evident or a part of the patient's problem.

D-13 Would require an endotracheal tube placement which has not yet been done. It would also be redundant.

	Possible	My Score
D-1	- 2	
D-2	+ 2	+2
D-3	+ 3	+3
D-4	- 2	
D-5	- 2	
D-6	+ 2	+2
D-7	- 2	-2
D-8	- 2	
D-9	0	
D-10	0	0
D-11	+ 2	
D-12	- 2	
D-13	- 1	
D-14	+ 1	+1
Total	**10**	6

SECTION C

Positive Scoring:

C-1 The arterial blood gases denote a patient in ventilatory failure. The values not only mandate intubation and ventilation, but mechanical ventilation when the patient is admitted and moved to an intensive care environment.

Negative Scoring:

C-2 Would be grievously harmful to the patient in the face of ventilatory failure.

C-3 Hyperinflation therapy, without an endotracheal tube, and on an ataxic patient is inappropriate.

C-4 Increasing the patient's precipitous oxygenation status would accomplish nothing towards reversing the ventilatory failure.

C-5 A bronchodilator is not indicated nor would its use on an ataxic patient be appropriate.

	Possible	My Score
C-1	+ 3	+3
C-2	- 3	
C-3	- 3	
C-4	- 3	
C-5	- 3	
Total	+ 3	+3

SECTION K

K-2 Is the optimal choice. Paralyzing the patient and controlling ventilation would solve the problems concomitant with an apneustic patient.

A diagram appears on pp. 835 of Burton and Hodgkins of the ataxic breathing pattern as well as other abnormal breathing patterns.

K-1 and K-4 Are scored positively as the need for mechanical ventilation was met. Both choices would be complicated by a highly irregular breathing pattern.

<u>Negative Scoring:</u>

K-3 Would provide insufficient tidal and minute volume for an 89 kg patient (12-15 ml/kg).

K-5 Requires spontaneous breathing which has been determined to be inadequate. Also at this point, we have no evidence of shunt, for which, PEEP is indicated.

	Possible	My Score
K-1	+ 1	+ 1
K-2	+ 3	
K-3	- 3	
K-4	+ 1	
K-5	- 3	
Total	+ 3	+ 1

SECTION H

Positive Scoring:

H-1 The IMV mode you chose was not successful. The patient's breathing pattern and ventilator "fighting", mandate paralyzing the patient and controlling ventilation.

Negative Scoring:

H-2, H-3, H-4, and H-5 Would all result in further deterioration of the patient, with disastrous results.

	Possible	My Score
H-1	+ 1	+1
H-2	- 3	
H-3	- 3	-3
H-4	- 3	
H-5	- 3	-3
Total	**+ 1**	-5

SECTIONG

Positive Scoring:

G-2 Is the preferable choice. By increasing rate and tidal volume, the patient, hopefully, would be placed in a moderate state of hyperventilation. Head trauma with concomitant intercranial pressure mandates a low CO_2 tension. The physiologic response is peripheral and cerebral vasoconstriction — of value to treat intracranial pressure/edema.

Negative Scoring:

G-1 Would not address the problem of increased intracranial pressure or hyperoxemia. As other medical means are available to treat intracranial pressure, it is scored at a lesser negative value.

G-3 As in G-1, the problem of intercranial pressure remains. This action would normalize acid base balance and oxygenation. Hence, the zero scoring.

G-4 and G-5 are inappropriate for control of CO_2 levels and an irregular breathing pattern.

	Possible	My Score
G-1	- 1	
G-2	+ 3	+3
G-3	0	
G-4	- 3	
G-5	- 3	
Total	+ 3	+3

SECTION B

Positive Scoring:

B-1 Is the preferable choice. It addresses the problem of shunt. The evidence for shunt is a decreased PO_2, and the x-ray results. The patient could be expected to elecit some manifestations of ARDS. The trauma itself could cause its onset. Head trauma is also a cause by itself due to massive sympathetic discharge. (Neurogenic pulmonary edema)

B-4 Is an acceptable response as it, also, addresses the problem of refractory shunt. It could upset the ideal PCO_2 that has been achieved. For that reason, it is scored at a lesser point value.

Negative Scoring:

B-2 Would ignore refractory shunt at the expense of maintaining an ideal PCO_2.

B-3 Not only is shunt refractory to increasing increments of FIO_2, but an 80% concentration adds the element of potential oxygen toxicity.

B-5 Would in no way contribute to solution of the patient's underlying problems.

	Possible	My Score
B-1	+ 3	+3
B-2	- 3	
B-3	- 3	
B-4	+ 1	
B-5	- 3	
Total	+ 3	+3

SECTION E

Positive Scoring:

E-1 Is the preferable choice. Discontinuance of intercranial pressure monitoring, paralyzing medication, the x-ray report, and an increasing compliance denote an improving patient. The question is, "Is he ready to be weaned?"

E-5 Is a viable, yet risky change. Because it is a step towards reducing hazards of positive pressure in the thorax, it is scored at a lesser positive score.

Negative Scoring:

E-2 This is a step in the wrong direction. A P_aO_2 of 84 mmHg is acceptable.

E-3 The patient is not ready to wean for the following reasons.

1. 10 cm H_2O PEEP is required to maintain a marginal P_aO_2.
2. Infiltrates are still present in the lung.
3. VD/VT is excessive.
4. % Shunt is excessive.
5. $(A\text{-}a)_{02}$ gradient.

E-4 Runs the risk of O_2 toxicity in the face of a satisfactory P_aO_2.

	Possible	My Score
E-1	+ 3	+3
E-2	- 3	
E-3	- 3	
E-4	- 3	
E-5	+ 2	
Total	+ 3	+3

JIM BURGEY

Route Possible	Scoring	My Score
A	+17	15
↓ F	+ 3	+3
↓ J	+ 3	+3
↓ D	+10	6
↓ C	+3	3
↓ K	+ 3	1
↘ H	+ 1	-5
↓ G	+ 3	+3
↓ B	+ 3	+3
↓ E	+ 3	+3
Total	48	35

Passing Score, Optimal Route 33
Alternate Route K, H, G 32

JIM BURGEY

REFERENCES

1. Burton, Hodgkins: **Respiratory Care a Guide to Clinical Practice, 2nd Edition,** Lippincott, 1984. (Pages 282-297, 648-651, 838-840)
2. Pilbeam: **Mechanical Ventilation Physiologic Applications and Clinical Applications,** Multi-Media Publishing, Inc., C.V. Mosby, 1986. (Pages 129-130)
3. Shapiro: **Clinical Application of Respiratory Care, 3rd Edition,** Year Book Medical Publishers, 1985. (Pages 62-68, 76-77, 393)

Walt Sampson

Clinical Simulation #7

Problem

WALT SAMPSON

You are a respiratory care person assigned to the cardiovascular intensive care unit of a 450-bed area medical center.

Mr. Sampson is a 66 year old male, with a diagnosis of myocardial infarction. He is being mechanically ventilated, SIMV mode, TV 850 ml, FIO_2 0.40, mandatory rate of 6/min. His arterial blood gases are pH 7.36, PCO_2 41 mmHg, PO_2 86 mmHg, HCO_3^- 21 mEq/l. There is a pulmonary artery catheter in place. He weighs 194 lbs. (88 kg).

NOW GO TO SECTION A

SECTION A

Data pertaining to Mr. Sampson is as follows:

- Spontaneous rate	15/min.	PCWP	21 mmHg
- Spontaneous TV	220 ml	PAP	42/24 mmHg
- Pulse	96/min.	CVP	12 mmHg
- Blood pressure	105/60 mm Hg	P_v0_2	33 mmHg
- Cardiac output	3.1 l/min.		

Chest x-rays reveal right lower lobe infiltrates. Breath sounds are diminished over the right lower lobe with scattered wheezing in that area.

Which would you recommend?

Choose only one, unless you are directed to "make another selection in this section".

A-1 Institute PEEP 5 cm H_2O

A-2 Institute postural drainage percussion and vibration Q4 hours

Physician agrees, go to Section J**

A-3 Administer acetylcysteine 10% Q4 hours

A-4 Increase TV to 1000 ml

A-5 Institute 2 sighs/hour of 1450 ml each

SECTION B

The defibrillation efforts are unsuccessful and the monitor tracing displays the following (below).

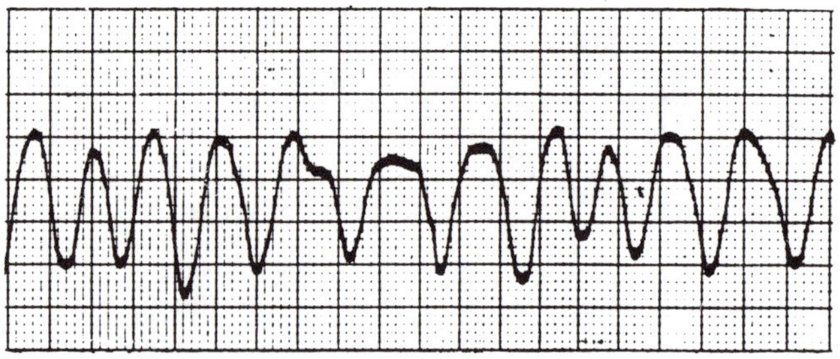

What would be your next course of action?

Choose only one, unless you are directed to "make another selection in this section".

B-1 Administer atropine IV	
B-2 Admini.;'er a precordial thump	
B-3 Administer bretylium toslate	
B-4 Administer lidocaine IV	
B-5 Administer cardiac compressions, ventilate with resuscitation bag FIO_2 1.0	Done, go to Section H**

SECTION C

The patient responds to therapy by converting to the tracing below.

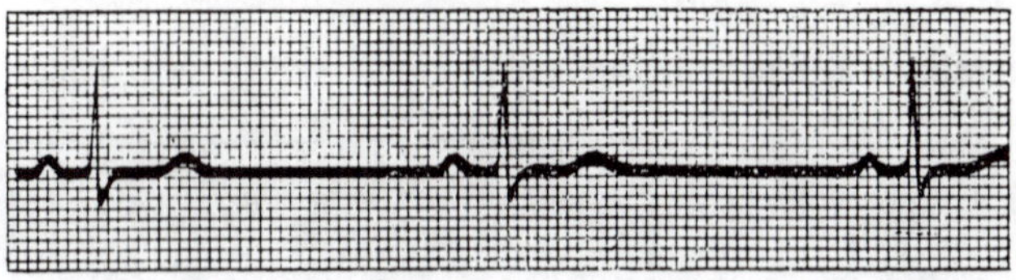

What would you recommend now?

Choose only one, unless you are directed to "make another selection in this section".

C-1 Administer atropine IV

C-2 Continue resuscitation per present protocol

C-3 Discontinue cardiac compressions

C-4 Extubate and place on esophageal obdurator

C-5 Discontinue manual ventilations. Replace on ventilator FIO_2 1.0, discontinue chest compression

SECTION D

Four hours later, ABG's are pH 7.41, PCO_2 41 mmHg, PCO_2 82 mmHg, HCO_3^- 23.5 mEq/l.

What would you recommend now?

Choose only one, unless you are directed to "make another selection in this section".

D-1 Maintain present parameters and monitor	
D-2 IMV rate 2, FIO_2 0.28, re-evaluate in 2 hours	
D-3 Discontinue mechanical ventilation, FIO_2 0.40 via T piece (Briggs adaptor) with heated aerosol	
D-4 Extubate, place on 40% venturi mask with aerosol	Done, end of problem
D-5 Extubate, place on nasal cannula, 4 lpm	

SECTION E

Based on the results of your evaluation, what would you recommend at this time?

Choose only one, unless you are directed to "make another selection in this section".

E-1 Maintain present parameters, re-evaluate in 12 hours

E-2 Decrease SIMV rate to 2/min. FIO_2 0.34, re-evaluate in 2 hours

E-3 CPAP mode, 5 cm H_20, FIO_2 0.40

E-4 Decrease TV to 600 ml FIO_2 0.30, re-evaluate in 12 hours

E-5 Remove from mechanical ventilation, place on T piece (Briggs) FIO_2 0.40 with heated aerosol

SECTION F

One hour later, Mr. Sampson is being mechanically ventilated in the assist/control mode, TV is 1000 ml, rate 10/ min., FIO_2 ABG's are pH 7.26, PCO_2 36 mmHg, PO_2 80 mmHg, HCO_3^- 15 mEq/l, B.E. -10. The ECG monitor tracing is below.

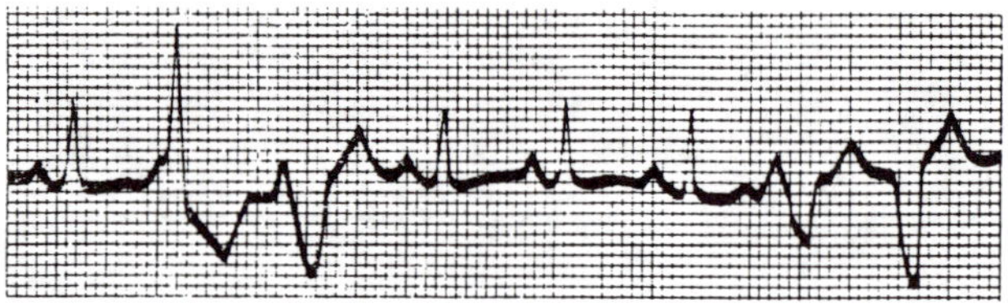

What would you recommend now?

Choose only one, unless you are directed to "make another selection in this section".

F-1 Administer verapamil

F-2 Administer epinephrine IV

F-3 Maintain present ventilator parameters. Administer sodium bicarbonate

Physician agrees, go to Section K.

F-4 Increase FIO_2 to 0.8

F-5 Administer atropine IV

SECTION G

After reconnecting the pulmonary artery catheter, you note the following tracing when the pulmonary capillary wedge pressure is recorded.

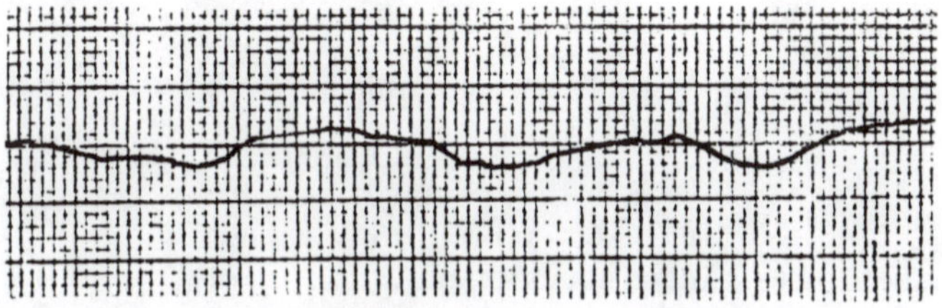

What would you recommend now?

Choose only one, unless you are directed to "make another selection in this section".

G-1	Continue present therapy and monitor	Physician disagrees, make another selection in this section.**
G-2	Request the physician to reposition the catheter tip	Done, go to Section F**
G-3	Place the patient in High Fowlers position	Physician disagrees, make another selection in this section.**
G-4	Retract the catheter tip 2-3 cm	Physician disagrees, make another selection in this section.**
G-5	Deflate the ballroom tip	Physician disagrees, make another selection in this section.**

SECTION H

After 4 minutes of cardiopulmonary resuscitation, lidocaine is being infused. Arterial blood gases are pH 7.18, PCO_2 58 mmHg, PO_2 68 mmHg, HCO_3^- 18.5 mEq/l, B.E. -11.

Which would you recommend now?

Choose only one, unless you are directed to "make another selection in this section".

H-1 Continue resuscitation per present protocol	Physician disagrees, make another selection in this section.**
H-2 Decrease FIO_2 to 0.50	
H-3 Administer atropine	
H-4 Administer sodium bicarbonate	Done, go to Section C.**
H-5 Instill epinephrine via the endotracheal tube	

SECTION I

Seven minutes into the resuscitation, the following ECG tracing is noted on the monitor. Lidocaine continues to be infused.

What would you recommend now?

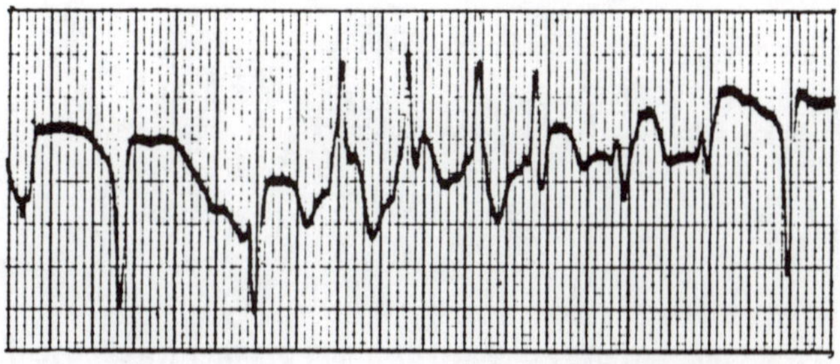

Choose only one, unless you are directed to "make another selection in this section".

I-1	Continue resuscitation per present protocol	Physician disagrees, make another selection in this
I-2	Administer bretylium toslate	Physician disagrees, make another selection in this
I-3	Replace on ventilator, FIO_2 1.0, monitor	Physician agrees, go to Section G**
I-4	Administer epinephrine via intracardiac needle	Physician disagrees, make another selection in this section.**
I-5	Administer atropine	

SECTION J

While positioning Mr. Sampson for his first treatment, you note a change in the ECG monitor pattern to that shown below.

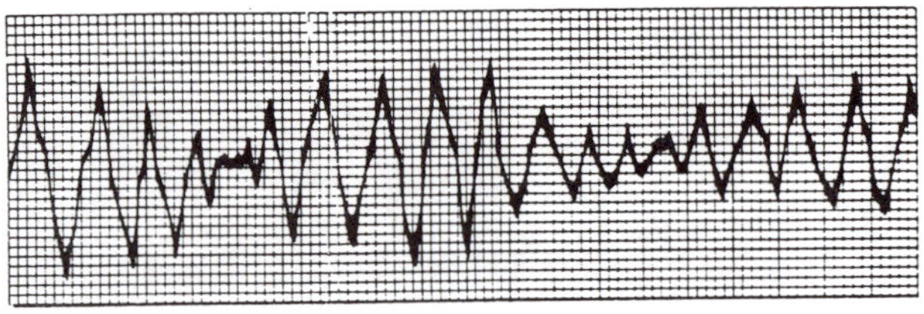

What would you do now?
Choose only one, unless you are directed to "make another selection in this section".

J-1 Administer one half ampule of sodium bicarbonate

J-2 Readjust the ECG monitor leads

J-3 Increase mandatory rate to 16/min., FIO_2 to 1.0

J-4 Press code alarm button, defibrillate at 350 Joules

J-5 Manually ventilate, FIO_2 1.0, begin cardiac compressions

SECTION K

Two days later you are asked to evaluate Mr. Sampson's pulmonary status.

Which would you choose?

Choose as many as you feel are indicated in this section.

K-1 CBC	Hb 13.5 gm%, Hct 38% WBC 7000 cm^3, RBC 4.8 cm^3**
K-2 Chest x-ray	Normal, ET tube properly placed **
K-3 Negative inspiratory force	-32 cm H_2O**
K-4 Carboxyhemoglobin level	
K-5 Urine pH	
K-6 Serum electrolytes	
K-7 Sensorium	Alert and oriented**
K-8 Ventilator parameters	SIMV rate 4/min. TV 1000 ml, FIO_2 0.4**
K-9 Sputum gram stain	Negligible pathogenic colonization**
K-10 Maximum voluntary ventilation	Not done**
K-11 Lactate level	
K-12 Vital signs	Pulse 82/min., blood pressure 120/70 mmHg, temp. 37.9 C**
K-13 Arterial blood gases	pH 7.42, PCO_2 38 mmHg, PO_2 89 mm Hg, HCO_3 24 mEq/l, %sat. 96%**
K-14 Estimated shunt (Q_s/Q_t)	11%**
K-15 V_d/V_t	32%**
K-16 Vital capacity	1600 ml**
K-17 Functional residual capacity	
K-18 Pupil reactivity	
K-19 **When you have completed your selections in this section, then develop K-19**	Go to Section E**

SECTION L

The ECG tracing remains unchanged.

What would you recommend now?

Choose only one, unless you are directed to "make another selection in this section".

L-1 Inject intracardiac epinephrine

L-2 Administer calcium gluconate

L-3 Administer cardiac compressions, ventilate with resuscitation bag FIO_2 1.0

L-4 Administer another precordial thump

L-5 Administer lidocaine

SECTION M

After thirty minutes, arterial blood gases are pH 7.33, PCO_2 47, PO_2 72, HCO_3^- 21, B.E. -2.

What would you recommend now?

Choose only one, unless you are directed to "make another selection in this section".

M-1 Increase PEEP to 10 cm H_2O, FIO_2 0.50	Physician disagrees, make another selection in this section.**
M-2 SIMV mode, rate 2/min. FIO_2 0.40, re-evaluate in 4 hours	Physician agrees, go to Section [illegible]**
M-3 Extubate, place on nasal cannula 4 lpm	Physician disagrees, make another selection in this section.**
M-4 Maintain present parameters, re-evaluate in 2 hours	Physician disagrees, make another selection in this section.**
M-5 Determine "Best" PEEP, adjust accordingly	Physician disagrees, make another selection in this section.**

Walt Sampson

Clinical Simulation #7

Answers, Explanations, and Scoring

WALT SAMPSON

This problem involves, primarily, the resuscitation of an arrested patient with underlying cardiac disease. It requires recognition of life threatening vs. non-life threatening arrythmias. Coincidentally, a problem is encountered with the pulmonary artery catheter. Finally, weaning from the ventilator must be considered.

SECTION A

Positive Scoring:

A-2 The scenario and additional information depicts a critical patient, at risk to interstitial and intrapulmonic pulmonary edema due to an elevated pulmonary capillary wedge pressure. Our patient, also, has underlying cardiac disease. Of all the choices offered, only one would materially contribute to the treatment of the patient—that being drainage of the infiltrate denoted by the x-ray.

Negative Scoring:

A-1 There is no evidence of shunt from the evidence at hand—shunt being the only indication for PEEP. Cardiac instability also obviates its use.

A-3 There is no evidence to warrant administration of a mucolytic.

A-4 The blood gas values are well within normal for a post MI patient. Increasing TV would materially harm the patient.

A-5 Sighs would be a means of preventing or correcting atelectasis, which is not evident from the information given. This modality is regional and controversial. It would be at the least, non-central to the treatment of the patient.

	Possible	My Score
A-1	- 3	
A-2	+ 3	+3
A-3	- 3	
A-4	- 3	
A-5	- 1	
Total	**+ 3**	+3

SECTION J

Positive Scoring:

J-4 Is immediately indicated. The rhythm strip is clearly, ventricular fibrillation. Immediate defibrillation is indicated and available in this clinical situation. Success at this juncture could eliminate, possibly, the need for further resuscitative measures.

Zero Scoring

J-5 Is the only other viable alternative. To commence ventilation and cardiac compressions would materially aid in survival of the patient—even if it was not the best alternative. It is forgiveable, and indicates recognition of the problem, at a lesser point value.

Negative Scoring:

J-1 Sodium bicarbonate is only, indicated after evidence of metabolic (lactic) acidosis has been established. It also would consume precious time at the expense of the patient's well-being.

J-2 Would be a time consuming search for ECG artifact in the face of ventricular fibrillation—of serious consequence to the patient.

J-3 Ventricular fibrillation is synonomous with cessation of cardiac output. Rate and FIO_2 do not substitute for lack of cardiac output. This action would be fatal to the patient in short time.

	Possible	My Score
J-1	- 3	
J-2	- 3	
J-3	- 3	
J-4	+ 3	+3
J-5	0	
Total	+3	+3

SECTION B

Positive Scoring:

B-5 Defibrillation is unsuccessful. Manual resuscitation is now in order. The patient has converted from coarse ventricular fibrillation to a more ominous, fine, pattern.

B-2 The precordial thump, although indicated in this monitored, witnessed situation, is to be used only when an electrical defibrillator is unavailable. The precordial thump, is rarely successful, and in non-fibrillatory arrythmias may precipitate ventricular fibrillation. This choice takes you into an alternate route.

Negative Scoring:

B-1 Is indicated for bradycardia only.

B-3 Bretylium toslate is indicated for ventricular ecopties which persist after lidocaine administration.

B-4 Lidocaine is indicated, but the priority is to establish cardiac output and ventilation/oxygenation. To not commence CPR could seriously harm the patient.

	Possible	My Score
B-1	- 3	
B-2	+ 1	
B-3	- 3	
B-4	- 3	
B-5	+ 2	+2
Total	**+ 2**	+2

ALTERNATE ROUTE
SECTION L

Positive Scoring:

L-3 The priority is to establish cardiac output and oxygenation. Initiate CPR!

Negative Scoring:

L-1 and L-5 May be indicated later in the resuscitation, but it is not the priority.

L-4 Precordial thump, if utilized, is indicated only on a "one thump" basis. More are contraindicated.

L-2 Calcium, at one time was used to treat asystole. It is no longer considered a first line therapy for "flatline", full arrest patients, and may actually, be counterproductive.

	Possible	My Score
L-1	- 3	
L-2	- 3	
L-3	+ 1	
L-4	- 3	
L-5	- 3	
Total	+ 1	

SECTION H

Positive Scoring:

H-4 Administer sodium bicarbonate. It is indicated as per the evidence of metabolic acidosis. The reversal of acidodis has priority over the administration of ino/chrono tropic drugs as these drugs are non-effecaceous in a low pH environment.

Zero Scoring:

H-5 Is scored zero as direct instillation of epinephrine into the endotracheal tube is indicated only, where intravenous routes are not yet available, or conditions exist that preclude intravenous lines — Because it could possibly be of benefit to the patient, you are not penalized for this choice.

Negative Scoring:

H-1 Ignores the problem of metabolic acidosis, but would mildly be detrimental to the patient.

H-2 Also ignores the problem of acidosis and could seriously harm the patient by precipitating additional acidosis.

H-3 Atropine is indicated only for bradycardia.

	Possible	My Score
H-1	- 1	-1
H-2	- 3	
H-3	- 3	
H-4	+ 3	+3
H-5	0	
Total	**+ 3**	+2

SECTION C

Positive Scoring:

C-1 Atropine is now indicated to treat sinus bradycardia. It would be central to the resolution of the patient's still potentially life threatening situation.

Zero Scoring:

C-2 Scores zero. It would sustain the patient, but would be non-contributory to solution of the immediate problem. It is forgiveable, but scores no points.

Negative Scoring:

C-3 The heart rate of 30 would be insufficient to maintain cardiac output. This action could seriously jeopardize the patient.

C-4 A move backward—potentially lethal.

C-5 Would accomplish ventilation, but would be counterproductive to cardiac output. The patient still requires chest compression to augment cardiac output.

	Possible	My Score
C-1	+ 3	+ 3
C-2	0	
C-3	- 3	
C-4	- 3	
C-5	- 3	
Total	**+ 3**	+3

SECTION I

Positive Scoring:

I-3 The tracing, multi-focal PVC's, indicated an effective rate of 60 beats/min. Marginal cardiac output is perfusing the patient. Replacement on the ventilator and careful monitoring is in order. Continued lidocaine therapy is specific for treatment of PVC's.

Negative Scoring:

I-1 Is now contraindicated. A chest compression on top of a T wave could put the heart back into a fibrillation status.

I-2 Is not indicated as the patient has responded to lidocaine.

I-4 Epinephrine could be of value to the heart due to its Beta 1 qualitities. The intracardiac route is contraindicated as the alternate routes are available. This procedure is also fraught with hazards and complications.

I-5 Is not indicated as a viable heart rhythm has been recaptured.

	Possible	My Score
I-1	- 3	-3
I-2	- 1	-1
I-3	+ 3	+3
I-4	- 3	-3
I-5	- 3	
Total	+ 3	-4

SECTION G

Positive Scoring:

G-2 The tracing indicates the tip of the catheter is wedged above the plane of the heart, and is recording alveolar pressure. By repositioning the tip below the plane of the heart, a true, static column of blood may be obtained.

Negative Scoring:

G-1 Failure to correct this problem would deprive the physician of vital information patient to the medical management of the patient.

G-3 Raising the patient to a near upright position would alter lung and cardiac hemodynamics.

G-4 Non-contributory to the resolution of the problem.

G-5 More of the same.

	Possible	My Score
G-1	- 2	-2
G-2	+ 3	+3
G-3	- 3	
G-4	- 3	-3
G-5	- 3	
Total	+ 3	-2

SECTION F

Positive Scoring:

F-3 The patient still elicits residual metabolic acidosis. The rhythm strip denotes a sinus rhythm typical of myocardial infarction. The solitary, unifocal PVC is typical in this class of patient. Therapy to eliminate acidosis is still indicated by pH, HCO_3^-, and -10 B.E.

Negative Scoring:

F-1 Verapamil is not indicated. It is a second line cardiac drug to treat supraventricular tachycardia.

F-2 The rate, and configuration of the tracing indicate sufficient cardiac output without the beta 1 adrenergic stimulating effects of epinephrine.

F-4 Not indicated! A PO_2 of 80 mmHg is near normal for a 66 year old man. It would not be harmful in the short run. Possibly harmful (O_2 toxicity) in the long run).

F-5 Not indicated. Sinus rate is 70/min. Bradycardia is usually defined as < 60/min.

	Possible	My Score
F-1	- 3	
F-2	- 3	
F-3	+ 3	+3
F-4	0	
F-5	- 3	
Total	**+ 3**	+3

SECTION K

Positive Scoring:

The emphasis on a ventilatory assessment of a patient with a non-intrapulmonic diagnosis should be weaning as soon as possible. Prolonged mechanical ventilation is fraught with serious complications.

K-2 Nothing is present to the preclude weaning.

K-3 Indicative of chest muscle strength sufficient to sustain spontaneous breathing.

K-6, K-7 Done daily on all intensive care patients.

K-8 SIMV rate of 4 indicates minimal support.

K-9 The patient has no residual infection.

K-12 Vital signs are within normals.

K-13 Arterial blood gases are favorable.

K-16 Vital capacity is approximately 18 ml/kg—favorable for weaning.

Zero Scoring:

K-1 and K-6 Are redundant. Their main contribution would be to run up the patient's bill.

K-14 and K-15 These are tests involving ventilation/perfusion abnormalities. This has never been a part of the problem.

K-18 Neither helpful, or harmful

Negative Scoring:
K-4 A test for carbon monoxide.
K-5, K-11 Of no value.
K-10 and K-17 Effort dependent. Difficult and usually involves moving the patient.

	Possible	My Score
K-1	- 2	-2
K-2	+ 3	+3
K-3	+ 1	+1
K-4	- 3	
K-5	- 3	
K-6	+ 1	
K-7	+ 1	+1
K-8	+ 2	+2
K-9	+ 1	+1
K-10	- 1	-1
K-11	- 2	
K-12	+ 1	+1
K-13	+ 2	+2
K-14	0	0
K-15	0	0
K-16	+ 2	+2
K-17	- 2	
K-18	0	
Total	+14	10

SECTION E

SECTION E

Positive Scoring:

E-5 All weaning parameters indicate the patient is ready to come off the ventilator. A "blitz" trial is warranted—with the ventilator at the bedside ready, if needed.

E-2 Is a more conservative approach, but understandable and still would contribute to the weaning effort at a lesser point value.

Negative Scoring:

E-1 and E-4 A 12 hour "wait and see" stance could jeopardize the patient to hazards and complications he doesn't need: infection, pneumothorax, decreased cardiac output, to name a few.

E-3 CPAP is not indicated. It would, also, upset a stable hemodynamic situation by placing additional positive pressure in the thorax. This choice directs you to alternate pathway.

	Possible	My Score
E-1	- 2	
E-2	+ 1	
E-3	- 1	
E-4	- 2	
E-5	+ 3	+3
Total	**+ 3**	+3

ALTERNATE ROUTE
SECTION M

Positive Scoring:

M-2 Is indicated as the ABG's indicate a retrogression of both acid/base and oxygenation status. The CPAP trial did not contribute to successful weaning of the patient. It was not disasterous, however.

Negative Scoring:

M-1, M-4, and M-5 Could all precipitate a further decline in the patient's status. Serious harm could befall the patient if these courses of action were instituted.

M-3 Would be a very rash action in the face of the deteriorating blood gases.

	Possible	My Score
M-1	- 3	
M-2	+ 1	
M-3	- 3	
M-4	- 3	
M-5	- 1	
Total	+ 1	

SECTION D

Positive Scoring:

D-4 Is now indicated, the patient has demonstrated adequacy of spontaneous ventilation to normalize acid base balance and to maintain satisfactory oxygenation.

D-2 and D-3 Are choices available to those who traversed an alternate route from Section M and scored at a less point value.

Negative Scoring:

D-1 Could prolong mechanical ventilation, or intubation unnecessarily, placing the patient at the concurrent risks of either situations. To protect the patient, the weaning and extubation should be accomplished as early as possible.

D-5 Extubation requires immediate, aerosol therapy, preferably heated treatment of glottic/subglottic edema is not provided by a nasal cannula.

	Possible	My Score
D-1	- 1	
D-2	+ 1	
D-3	+ 2	
D-4	+ 3	+3
D-5	- 2	
Total	**+ 3**	+3

WALT SAMPSON

Route	Scoring: Possible	Scoring: My Score
A	+3	+3
J	+3	+3
B	+2	+2
L	+1	
H	+3	+2
C	+3	+3
I	+3	-4
G	+3	-2
F	+3	+3
K	+14	+10
E	+3	+3
M	+1	0
D	+3	+3
TOTAL	43	26

FAIL

Optimal Route Passing Score **30**
All alternate routes **29**

REFERENCES

1. Burton, Hodgkins: **Respiratory Care a Guide to Clinical Practice, 2nd Edition,** Lippincott, 1984. (Pages 282-287, 648-651)

2. JAMA: **Part III Adult Advanced Cardiac Life Support, Volume 255, No. 21,** June 1986. (Pages 2933-2951)

3. Pilbeam: **Mechanical Ventilation Physiologic Applications and Clinical Applications,** Multi-Media Publishing, Inc., C.V. Mosby, 1986. (Pages 163-205, 273-296)

4. Shapiro: **Clinical Application of Respiratory Care, 3rd Edition,** Year Book Medical Publishers, 1985. (Pages 297-311, 313-325, 372-378).PA

Janice Wills

Clinical Simulation #8

Problem

JANICE WILLS

SCENARIO

You are a respiratory therapist in a 650-bed county hospital. The charge nurse of the neurology service calls you for a respiratory consult on Janice Wills, a newly admitted patient. She is a 33 year old housewife with a history of Myesthenia Gravis. She weighs 112 pounds (51 kg) and is 5'5" in height.

NOW GO TO SECTION A

SECTION A

Mrs. Wills' chart reveals a hospitalization two years previous with the same diagnosis. Since that time she has been on a regimen of prostigmine. The present admission was precipitated by extreme shortness of breath on minimal exertion.

For a preliminary assessment of the patient, which would you choose?

Choose as many as you feel are indicated in this section.

A-1 Functional residual capacity	Not done**
A-2 Chest auscultation	Diminished, equal, bilaterally.**
A-3 Arterial blood gases	pH 7.39, PCO_2 43 mmHg, PO_2 89 mmHg, HCO_3 26 mEq/l, FIO_2 0.21**
A-4 Past medical history	Non-remarkable excepting Myesthenia Gravis history**
A-5 General appearance	Listless, eyelids drooping**
A-6 FEV_1/FVC %	55%, performed with difficulty**
A-7 Muscle tone	Facial ptosis (drooping)**
A-8 Gag reflex	Present**
A-9 Smoking history	
A-10 Vital capacity	
A-11 Heart sounds	
A-12 Bowel sounds	
A-13 Babinski reflex	
A-14 Breathing pattern	
A-15 Deep tendon reflex	
A-16 Tidal volume	
A-17 Sputum production	

A-18 Vital signs

A-19 When you have completed your selections in this section, then develop A-19

SECTION B

Which would you now recommend?

Choose only one, unless you are directed to "make another selection in this section."

B-1 Institute mask CPAP 5 cm H_20

B-2 Institute postural drainage, percussion and vibration Q4 hours

B-3 Intubate and ventilate

B-4 Institute oxygen therapy, 28% venturi mask

B-5 Bronchodilator therapy Albuterol 4 mg, Q4 hours

SECTION C

One hour later, the arterial blood gas results are: pH 7.31, PCO_2 52 mmHg, PO_2 88 mmHg, HCO_3^- 26 mEq/l Mrs. Wills' respiratory rate is 24/min., tidal volume is 280 ml, blood pressure is 140/110 mmHg.

Which of the following would you recommend?

Choose only one, unless you are directed to "make another selection in this section."

C-1 Intubate. Support ventilation via resuscitation bag rate 12/min.

C-2 Decrease FIO_2 to 0.28

C-3 Discontinue oxygen therapy

C-4 Support ventilation FIO_2 1.0. Transfer to intensive care unit

C-5 Intubate. CPAP 10 cm H_2O FIO_2 0.28

SECTION D

Two weeks later, Mrs. Wills remains mechanically ventilated (7200 Puritan Bennett). She was treated, successfully, for two bouts of gram (-) pulmonary sepsis, but remains unable to sustain adequate, spontaneous ventilation. Data is as follows:

Ventilator	Patient
Tidal volume 700 ml	ABG's pH 7.45, PCO_2 38 mmHg,
SIMV Rate 12/min.	PO_2 100 mmHg, HCO_3^- 25 mEq/l
Spontaneous rate 6/min.	Blood pressure 98/50 mmHg
FIO_2 0.30	Temperature 38 C
Flow rate 22 lpm	Pulse 84/min.
Peak pressure 30 cm H_2O	Urine output 1100 ml/24 hrs
Plateau Pressure 0.5 sec.	
I:E ratio 1:1.1	
Mean airway pressure 14 cm H_2O	

What ventilator changes would you recommend?

Choose only one, unless you are directed to "make another selection in this section."

D-1 Tidal volume 800 ml SIMV rate 14, flow rate 24 lpm, plateau pressure 0.5 sec.

D-2 Tidal volume 650 ml, SIMV rate 6, flow rate 18 lpm, plateau pressure off.

D-3 Pressure support 10 cm H_2O

D-4 Control mode, Tidal volume 650 ml, SIMV rate 12, flow rate 22 lpm

SECTION E

24 Hours later, beginning your shift in the intensive care unit, Mrs. Wills' ventilator parameters and data are as follows:

Ventilator

Tidal volume 650 ml
SIMV Rate 10/min.
Spontaneous rate 0
FIO_2 0.30
Flow rate 18 lpm
Peak pressure 28 cm H_2O
I:E ratio 1:3
Mean airway pressure 8 cm H_2O

Patient

ABG's pH 7.38, PCO_2 39 mmHg
PO_2 96 mmHg, HCO_3^- 24 meQ/l
Blood pressure 115/72 mmHg
Temperature 38° C
Urine output 1100 ml/24 hrs

While working with another patient, you hear Mrs. Wills' ventilator alarming. The display denotes the cause to be improper I:E ratio. To correct this problem, which would you evaluate?

Choose as many as you wish in this section.

E-1 High pressure alarm setting	
E-2 FIO_2 Setting	
E-3 Plateau pressure	
E-4 Tidal volume	
E-5 Rate	
E-6 Kinking of endotracheal tube	
E-7 Peak pressure	
E-8 Static Compliance	
E-9 Flow rate control	
E-10 When you have completed your selections in this section, then develop E-10**	

SECTION F

Which would you recommend at this time?

Choose only one, unless you are directed to "make another selection in this section."

F-1 Aerosol therapy — via USN .5 normal saline

Physician disagrees, make another selection in this section.**

F-2 Hyperinflation therapy (IPPB) QID with normal saline

Physician disagrees, make another selection in this section.**

F-3 Forced vital capacity and tidal volume Q2 hours

Physician agrees, go to Section I**.

F-4 Complete pulmonary function (spirometry, volumes, capacities, D_LCO)

Physician disagrees, make another selection in this section.**

F-5 Exercise stress test utilizing Bruce protocol

Physician disagrees, make another selection in this section.**

SECTION G

Four hours later, Mrs. Wills' vital capacity is 350 ml. She states she is experiencing difficulty swallowing.

What would you do now?

Choose only one, unless you are directed to "make another selection in this section."

G-1 Place patient in high Fowlers position. Notify the attending physician.

G-2 Instruct the patient to take deepest breath possible.

G-3 Increase the FIO_2 to 0.5

G-4 Reassure Mrs. Wills that this is normal for her condition.

G-5 Increase the FIO_2 to 1.0

SECTION H

The resident assigned to Mrs. Wills is concerned she will contact a nosocomial infection. He requests your recommendations on measures that would prevent this situation from happening — or to speed the response time if infection were to occur.

Which would you recommend?

Choose as many as you wish in this section.

H-1 Administer a broad spectrum antibiotic daily	Physician disagrees, not done**
H-2 Graph static compliance Q2 hours	Done**
H-3 Maintain in high Fowlers position	Done**
H-4 Oropharyngeal culture daily	Done**
H-5 Stomach content pH daily	Done, pH maintained at <4.0**
H-6 Place in protective isolation	Not done**
H-7 VD/VT % daily	Not done**
H-8 Maintain I:E ratio at 1:2	Not done**
H-9 Maintain "no leak" cuff pressure	Done, Cuff maintained at 25 cm H_2O**
H-10 Place condensate traps in in ventilator circuitry (inspiratory and expiratory limbs)	Done**
H-11 Personnel to wash hands before touching patient	Done**
H-12 Change ventilator circuitry Q24 hours	
H-13 Substitute heat-moisture exchanger (artificial nose) for ventilator humidifier	
H-14 Change endotracheal tubes Q3 days	
H-15 Measure oxygen uptake (V_{02}) daily	
H-16 Babinski reflex test Q4 hours	
H-17 Gram stain of tracheal aspirate daily	
H-18 <u>When</u> you have <u>completed</u> your selections in this section, then <u>develop H-18</u>	

SECTION I

24 Hours after admission, Mrs. Wills' vital capacity is 1.2 liters. She states she feels very short of breath. The attending physician asks your assistance in further evaluation of the patient.

Which would you recommend?

Choose as many as you feel are indicated in this section.

I-1 Sputum production

I-2 ECG

I-3 Serum electrolytes

I-4 Arterial blood gases

I-5 Pulmonary artery pressure

I-6 Chest x-ray

I-7 Shunt study
100% oxygen $(A - a)_{O2}$
difference

I-8 Dysphagia
(difficulty swallowing)

I-9 Chest auscultation

I-10 Diaphragmatic breathing exercises

I-11 Tidal volume

I-12 Diagnostic chest percussion

I-13 Respiratory rate and pattern

I-14 Range of motion

I-15 Venous % saturation

I-16 Static compliance

I-17 Lactic acid level

I-18 Level of consciousness

I-19 Airways resistance (Raw)

I-20 <u>When</u> you have <u>completed</u> your selections in this section, then <u>develop I-20</u>

SECTION J

The physician arrives and requests a "stat" blood gas. Values are pH 7.34, PCO_2 47 mmHg, PO_2 55 mmHg, HCO_3^- 25 mEq/l. He administers an increased dosage of prostigmine and asks you to obtain another arterial blood gas in one hour and report back to him.

What action would you recommend pending results of this test?

Choose only one, unless you are directed to "make another selection in this section."

J-1 Increase FIO_2 to 35% via venturi mask	Physician agrees, go to Section C**
J-2 Maintain present therapy. Monitor	Physician disagrees, make another selection in this section.**
J-3 Intubate - Institute Mask CPAP 5 cm H_2O, FIO_2 0.40	Physician disagrees, make another selection in this section.**
J-4 Aerosol therapy. Ultrasonic nebulizer, FIO_2 0.35	Done, go to Section C**
J-5 Oxygen therapy via partial rebreather mask	Physician agrees, go to Section C**

SECTION K

Twenty minutes later, arterial blood gases are pH 7.46, PCO_2 37 mmHg, PO_2 37 mmHg, PO_2 110 mmHg, HCO_3^- 24 mEq/l.

On the basis of this information, which ventilator settings would you choose?

Choose only one, unless you are directed to "make another selection in this section."

K-1 Rate 6/min., tidal volume 50 ml FIO_2 0.30

K-2 Rate 14/min. Tidal volume 950 ml, FIO_2 0.50

K-3 CPAP mode, 5 cm H_2O, FIO_2 0.30

K-4 Rate 8/min. Tidal volume 700 ml, PEEP 5 cm H_2O

K-5 Rate 10/min. Tidal volume 700 ml, FIO_2 0.30

SECTION L

Fifteen minutes later the spontaneous tidal volume is 275 ml. The patient's pulse is 124/minute and "thready".

What would you recommend now?

Choose only one, unless you are directed to "make another selection in this section."

L-1 Increase rate of ventilation to 14/minute	Physician disagrees, make another selection in this section.**
L-2 Place on Bird Mark 7 ventilator - assist mode	Physician disagrees, make another selection in this section.**
L-3 Transfer immediately to an intensive care unit. FIO_2 0.1	Physician agrees, go to Section M**
L-4 Place on PR 2 Bennett ventilator - assist mode	Physician disagrees, make another selection in this section.**
L 5 Maintain present therapy Monitor	Physician disagrees, make another selection in this section.**

SECTION M

On arrival in the intensive care unit, the patient is intubated and placed on a Puritan Bennett 7200 ventilator. The resident on duty asks your recommendations for initial ventilator parameters.

Which would you choose?

Choose only one, unless you are directed to "make another selection in this section."

M-1 Control mode, rate 10,
Tidal volume 450 ml,
FIO_2 0.5, PEEP 5 cm H_2O

M-2 SIMV mode, rate 10,
Tidal volume 600 ml
FIO_2 0.30

M-3 SIMV mode, rate 12,
Tidal volume 850 ml,
FIO_2 0.4

M-4 Assist/Control mode,
Machine rate 10,
Tidal volume 600 ml, FIO_2 0.3

M-5 Control mode, rate 12,
Tidal volume 850 ml,
5 cm H_2O PEEP, FIO_2 0.4

Janice Wills

Clinical Simulation #8

Answers, Explanations, and Scoring

JANICE WILLS

The patient is a progressively deteriorating Myesthenia Gravis. You are required to manage her course of treatment. This involves evaluation, close monitoring, ventilator commitment, and measures to protect the patient from nosocomial infection. You are also required to solve problems involving I:E ratio and the effects of positive pressure in the thorax.

THE SCENARIO

You are presented with a case involving neurologic disease which has progressed to the point of restrictive pulmonary inpairment. The character of myesthenia Gravis is a disease of gradual swings, both upward and downward. As the muscles of ventilation weaken, hypoventilation may progress to ventilatory failure. Treatment with an anti-acytelcholinergic drug (prostigmine) is hazardous in that overadministration creates a situation similar to the disease itself—inability of the motor nerve impulse to quickly traverse the synapse.

The cause of the disease is unknown. When ventilatory failure occurs, treatment is mechanical ventilation until the condition decides to improve. This may be rapidly, or prolonged for months. During these periods, the patient is at risk to the severe hazards of intubation, mechanical ventilation (positive pressure), nosocomial infection, and human error.

The principal neurologic diseases (m. Gravis and Guillain-Barre) are discussed on pp. 837 of Burton and Hodgkins.

This problem would also apply to:

- Spinal cord injury causing chest muscle paralysis
- Poliomyelitis
- Landry's ascending paralysis
- Tick bite paralysis
- Muscular dystrophy
- Tetanus

SECTION A

<u>Positive Scoring:</u>

A-2 Auscultation would provide a baseline for ongoing assessment of audible adequacy of ventilation.

A-3 ABG's are central to quantifying the degree of ventilatory impairement.

A-5, A-7 Are helpful as they, also, are outward symptoms of the disease.

A-9 Is of marginal value, but still, a factor to consider for possible pulmonary complications.

A-10 Vital capacity is central to the assessment of, and serial tracking of the disease process.

A-4 and A-14 An important element of a pulmonary assessment.

A-16 An important parameter when compared to vital capacity. When the two are equal there is no ventilatory reserve.

A-18 Are relevant baselines.

Zero Scoring:

A-6 and A-17 Are irrelevant, but would neither help nor harm the patient.

Negative Scoring:

A-1 Would be time consuming and foregone conclusion.

A-8, A-13, and A-15 Are tests which are redundant and inflict pain on the patient.

A-11 and A-12 Are outside the scope of a pulmonary assessment.

	Possible	My Score
A-1	- 2	
A-2	+ 1	
A-3	+ 3	
A-4	+ 1	
A-5	+ 2	
A-6	0	
A-7	+ 2	
A-8	- 2	
A-9	+ 1	
A-10	+ 3	
A-11	- 2	
A-12	- 2	
A-13	- 2	
A-14	+ 2	
A-15	- 1	
A-16	+ 2	
A-17	0	
A-18	+ 1	
Total	**18**	

SECTION F

Positive Scoring:

F-3 From the assessment completed in Section A, we know the patient is in jeopardy to ventilatory failure but, as yet has adequate ventilation (PCO_2 43 mmHg).

A serial measurement of forced vital capacity at the bedside is the easiest, cheapest, yet accurate means of monitoring the ventilatory reserves available to the patient.

Negative Scoring:

F-1 There is no evidence of indications for aerosol therapy at present.

F-2 IPPB also is not indicated. It too has risks involved. It has no value towards resolution of the patient's immediate problem.

F-4 These tests are redundant as well as expensive and involve effort dependency. We already know the problem's etiology.

F-5 Although a past medical history could possibly yield a pertinent fact, we know all factors which pertain to a respiratory assessment. It would be redundant and a waste of time.

	Possible	My Score
F-1	- 3	
F-2	- 2	
F-3	+ 3	
F-4	- 3	
F-5	- 2	
Total	+ 3	

SECTION I

Positive Scoring:

Central to the scoring of this section is that the patient has healthy lungs. The problem is restrictive pulmonary disease secondary to neurologic impairment of the ventilatory pump.

I-4 ABG's are central to assessing adequacy of ventilation (PCO_2).

I-8 Difficulty swallowing is a symptom of myesthenia Gravis and a precursor of aspiration.

I-9 Auscultation, easily accomplished, verifies the degree of air movement in and out of the lung.

I-11 and I-13 Central to adequacy of ventilation, 350 ml is the lower limit of normal. The patient is compensating by rapid, shallow breathing.

I-18 Mild confusion is an indicator of early hypoxemia.

Zero Scoring:

I-2 There is no evidence of cardiac arrythmia. It would neither help or harm the patient.

Negative Scoring:

I-1 There is no evidence of pulmonary infection.

I-5, I-7, I-15, and I-19 Require pulmonary artery cannulation — not in place.

I-3, I-6, I-12, and I-19 Are either redundant or not in the scope of respiratory care.

I-10 and I-14 Are rehabilitation procedures.

I-16 and I-17 Not appropriate for this patient.

	Possible	My Score
I-1	- 1	
I-2	0	
I-3	- 2	
I-4	+ 3	
I-5	- 2	
I-6	- 1	
I-7	- 2	
I-8	+ 2	
I-9	+ 1	
I-10	- 2	
I-11	+ 2	
I-12	- 2	
I-13	+ 2	
I-14	- 2	
I-15	- 2	
I-16	- 2	
I-17	- 2	
I-18	+ 1	
I-19	- 2	
Total	11	

SECTION B

B-4 The patient is hypoxemic. Treatment is supplemental oxygen therapy. The underlying cause being hypoventilation. It is now obvious the patient is in early ventilatory failure. If she deteriorates further it will become acute ventilatory failure.

Negative Scoring:

B-1 Would require spontaneous breathing and adequate muscle strength — lacking in our patient.

B-2 There are no indications present for postural drainage.

B-3 Intubation and ventilation are possibilities but premature. It is possible the patient is at the bottom of their downswing, or might respond to prostigmine therapy and avoid this hazardous procedure.

B-5 Bronchodilator therapy is redundant as there is no evidence of bronchoconstriction.

	Possible	My Score
B-1	- 3	
B-2	- 3	
B-3	- 3	
B-4	+ 3	
B-5	- 3	
Total	+ 3	

SECTION G

Positive Scoring:

G-1 The patient's vital capacity has dropped to the point it equals tidal volume. This is a very ominus situation as there is no ventilatory reserve. Immediate, positive action is necessary. Medicating and transferring a critical patient is beyond the scope of respiratory practice — notifying a physician of an ominus situation is.

Placing the patient upright as possible is for the prevention of aspiration — a distinct possibility.

Negative Scoring:

G-2 and G-4 Are of no help. She cannot breathe deeply and presumably, she knows the finer details of her diagnosis.

G-3 and G-5 Might possibly be of some benefit to correct her hypoxemia, but would be offset by failing to address the deteriorating acid base balance, which became evident on the last blood gas values.

	Possible	My Score
G-1	+ 3	
G-2	- 3	
G-3	- 3	
G-4	- 3	
G-5	- 3	
Total	+ 3	

SECTION J

Positive Scoring:

J-1 and J-5 Both score positively. The results of the prostigmine trial would not be affected. Oxygen would be a palliative measure pending assessment of the increased prostigmine trial. With acidosis and a low PO_2, hypoxia may, safely be assumed. Prevention of unacceptable tissue oxygenation is appropriate and in the best interest of the patient.

Negative Scoring:

J-2 Is unacceptable as the respiratory status trend is downward. To do nothing could cause the patient serious harm.

J-3 CPAP requires spontaneous breathing, in which the patient has demonstrated inadequacy.

J-4 No indications exist for aerosol therapy. Because it does include supplemental oxygen, it is scored at a lesser, negative value.

	Possible	My Score
J-1	+ 3	
J-2	- 3	
J-3	- 3	
J-4	- 1	
J-5	+ 3	
Total	+ 3	

SECTION C

Positive Scoring:

C-4 Is the preferable answer. The prostigmine trial failed and the patient is in acute ventilating failure (PCO_2 > 50 mmHg, PO_2 < 50 mmHg). The patient faces long term mechanical ventilation — The only appropriate place for which is an intensive care setting.

C-1 Is acceptable, but fails to address the need for close monitoring, visual surveillance and other considerations provided by an intensive care unit. This choice directs you on an alternate route at a lesser point value.

Negative Scoring:

C-2, C-3, and C-5 Would all be disasterous in the face of ventilatory failure.

	Possible	My Score
C-1	+ 1	
C-2	- 3	
C-3	- 3	
C-4	+ 3	
C-5	- 3	
Total	+3	

ALTERNATE ROUTE
SECTION L

Positive Scoring:

L-3 The patient continues to deteriorate as indicated by the diminishing tidal volume. At this point, there should be no doubt the patient will be requiring mechanical ventilatory support. This mandates an intensive care setting.

Negative Scoring:

L-1 and L-5 This would support the patient, but practicability dictates this to be a futile course.

L-2 and L-4 Both ventilators require continuous monitoring by a therapist. In most hospitals, this course of action would violate the procedure manual — mechanical ventilation is done only in an intensive care unit.

	Possible	My Score
L-1	- 3	
L-2	- 3	
L-3	+ 1	
L-4	- 3	
L-5	- 3	
Total	**+ 1**	

SECTION M

Positive Scoring:

M-2 and M-4 Are choices demonstrating the similarities of assist/control and SIMV. Both would be a comfortable mode for a patient spontaneously breathing. Also, both would sustain the patient in the event of apnea — a possibility.

The salient point is that a satisfactory tidal volume is calculated (12-15 ml/kg).

M-3 While outside the norms for initial tidal volume it is forgiveable, but at a lesser score. It takes you on an alternate route.

Negative Scoring:

M-1 and M-5 Are erronious for several reasons. Tidal volumes are inaccurate. FIO_2's excessively high for a patient with normal lungs. Most importantly, PEEP is not indicated.

	Possible	My Score
M-1	- 3	
M-2	+ 3	
M-3	+ 1	
M-4	+ 3	
M-5	- 3	
Total	+ 3	

SECTION K

Positive Scoring:

K-5 An accurate assessment of the blood gases should lead you to diminution of tidal volume and FIO_2. To not proceed on this course could cause the patient serious harm.

Negative Scoring:

K-1 Does not meet accepted criteria for minute volume or tidal volume. (TV 12-15ml/kg)

K-2 Does not meet accepted criteria for minute volume or tidal volume either.

K-3 Is unacceptable for a hypoventilating patient.

K-4 There is no evidence of presence of indications for PEEP.

	Possible	My Score
K-1	- 3	
K-2	- 3	
K-3	- 3	
K-4	- 3	
K-5	+ 1	
Total	**+ 1**	

SECTION H

Positive Scoring:

H-2 Yes. A downtrend of compliance is a precursor to respiratory infection. An early warning is of benefit.

H-3 Yes. Retrograde flow of condensate is associated with "washing" of colonized bacteria into the patient's lungs.

H-4 Heavy oropharyngeal colonization is associated with nosocomial pneumonias. This, also, could provide early warning of danger.

H-5 Heavy dosage of antiacid is associated with colonization by pathogens when pH rises above 4.0. Aspiration of infected stomach contents is a major source of nosocomial pneumonias.

H-9 Yes. This would aid in preventing colonized secretions from reaching the lung.

H-10 Yes. This relates to H-3 and the possibility of retrograde flow of ventilator tubing condensate.

H-11 A very basic, effective method.

H-12 Daily changes of circuitry would be of help, particularly when normal procedure is for change Q48 hours.

H-14 The heaviest colonization of pathogens is on the inner surfaces of the tube. Frequent change would be of benefit.

H-17 Yes. This would provide the earliest warning that infection was present.

Zero Scoring:

H-6 Although possibly beneficial, is expensive, cumbersome, and is reserved for immunosuppressed, severely compromised patients.

Negative Scoring:

H-1 Would be the means for normal flora to become "fast", and pathogenic.

H-7, H-8, H-15, and H-16 Would have no benefit in protecting the patient from nosocomial infection.

H-13 Heat-moisture exchangers are associated with humidity deficits and plugging. Both would be harmful, if they occurred. There is no point in risking these hazards.

	Possible	My Score
H-1	- 2	
H-2	+ 1	
H-3	+ 2	
H-4	+ 2	
H-5	+ 2	
H-6	0	
H-7	- 1	
H-8	- 1	
H-9	+ 2	
H-10	+ 2	
H-11	+ 2	
H-12	+ 2	
H-13	- 2	
H-14	+ 2	
H-15	- 2	
H-16	- 1	
H-17	+ 2	
Total	**19**	

SECTION E

Please note you are given data really not relevant to the immediate problem of improper I:E ratio. This is "bridge" information which will be necessary to make your choices in the succeeding section.

Positive Scoring:

E-4, E-5, E-6, E-7, and E-8 Are all factors which, if inadvertant, or if a "knob twister" changed settings without telling anyone, could cause the I:E ratio to alarm.

E-9 The most likely source, as the latent image answer proves, has fallen victim to someone slowing the flow to where inspiratory time exceeds expiratory time. This would be understandable in a large, county, teaching hospital.

Negative Scoring:

E-1 and E-2 Would have no bearing on I:E ratio.

E-3 If extended, would lengthen expiratory time — which has a limit. It would not alarm even if extended to the limit.

	Possible	My Score
E-1	- 1	
E-2	- 1	
E-3	- 1	
E-4	+ 2	
E-5	+ 2	
E-6	+ 2	
E-7	+ 2	
E-8	+ 2	
E-9	+ 2	
Total	**12**	

SECTION D

By examining the data in the preceding section, you should note a pronounced drop in urine output and blood pressure. These are classic responses to long term ventilator commitment and, concomitant, positive pressure in the thorax. Your choice should be one which results in lowered, mean airway pressure.

Positive Scoring:

D-2 On a volume ventilator, mean airway pressure is directly proportional to several factors. Lowering tidal volume, reducing machine rate, shortening inspiratory time, and eliminating plateau pressure would all contribute to reducing mean airway pressure.

By increasing the flow rate (14 to 18 lpm) the I:E ratio would be increased to approximately 1:1.2.

Negative Scoring:

D-1 Would worsen the situation by increasing mean airway pressure.

D-3 Is a weaning procedure. There is no evidence the patient is ready for, or in a weaning mode.

D-4 Would only partially address the problem of mean airway pressure by decreasing inspiratory time, and decreasing tidal volume.

	Possible	My Score
D-1	- 3	
D-2	+ 3	
D-3	- 3	
D-4	- 1	
Total	**+1**	

JANICE WILLS

ROUTE	SCORING: Possible	SCORING: My Score
A	17	
F	3	
I	11	
B	+ 3	
G	+ 3	
J	+ 3	
C	+3 +1	
L	+ 1	
M	+3 +1	
K	+1	
H	19	
E	12	
D	3	
Total	**80**	

Optimal Route Passing Score **54**
Alternate Route Passing Score **55**

JANICE WILLS

REFERENCES

1. Burton, Hodgkins: **Respiratory Care a Guide to Clinical Practice, 2nd Edition,** Lippincott, 1984. (Pages 452-454, 567, 836, 837, 844-848)

2. Pilbeam: **Mechanical Ventilation Physiologic Applications and Clinical Applications,** Multi-Media Publishing, Inc., C.V. Mosby, 1986. (Pages 130-132, 141, 142, 224-226)

3. Shapiro: **Clinical Application of Respiratory Care, 3rd Edition,** Year Book Medical Publishers, 1985. (Pages 541 and 542).

James Wilson

Clinical Simulation #9

Problem

JAMES WILSON

You are a respiratory therapist working the p.m. shift in your 225-bed community hospital. At 9:30 p.m. you are paged to the emergency room to assist with the care of James Wilson. He is a 3 1/2 year old male. After being introduced to James and his parents, you note he is extremely hoarse and breathing with difficulty. There is no emergency room physician on staff.

NOW GO TO SECTION A

SECTION A

After commencing oxygen and aerosol therapy on James, and pending arrival of the attending physician, which would you assess?

Choose as many as you feel are indicated in this section.

A-1 Medical History

A-2 Urinalysis

A-3 Temperature

A-4 Pupillary response

A-5 FEV_1/FVC %

A-6 Respiratory rate and pattern

A-7 Throat culture

A-8 Onset of present illness

A-9 Flow/volume loop studies

A-10 Diagnostic chest percussion

A-11 Breath sounds

A-12 Residual volume and functional Residual Volume (FRC)

A-13 Chest inspection

A-14 General appearance

A-15 CBC and differential

A-16 **When you have completed your selections in this section, then develop A-16**

SECTION B

Based on the information gathered in the previous section, what would be the most likely cause of James' present condition?

Choose only one, unless you are directed to "make another selection in this section".

B-1 Bronchiolitis

B-2 Cystic Fibrosis

B-3 Laryngotracheobronchitus (Croup)

B-4 Epiglottitis

B-5 Pertussis (whooping cough)

SECTION C

The attending pediatrician arrives. She asks for your recommendations on tests to determine the specific cause of James' respiratory problem.

Choose as many as you feel are indicated in this section.

C-1 Chest x-ray	Ordered—Normal**
C-2 Spinal tap	Not done**
C-3 Review of CBC results	Hct 43% Hb 14.6% WBC 13,000**
C-4 Review of throat culture	Heavy colonization of gram(-) rods**
C-5 Fluid challenge	Not done**
C-6 Ability to swallow	Cannot swallow**
C-7 Diffusion of the lung (D_LCO)	Not done**
C-8 Lateral neck x-ray	Ordered; marked soft tissue edema, glottic area**
C-9 Visual exam of glottis and epiglottis	Swollen, red epiglottis and glottic area**
C-10 Arterial blood gases	Ordered—pH 7.36, PCO_2 45 mmHg, PO_2 85 mmHg, HCO_3 23 mEq/l**
C-11 **When you have completed your selections in this section, then develop C-11**	Go to Section D**

SECTION D

The attending physician agrees with your conclusions as to James' condition. She now asks for your recommendations as to a course of action to treat James.

Which would you recommend?

Choose as many as you feel are indicated in this section.

D-1 Cool mist tent. O_2 at 15 lpm	
D-2 Observe closely for increasing respiratory distress	
D-3 Institute postural drainage, percussion and vibration Q2 hours	
D-4 Alert on-call surgeon and anesthesiologist for possible tracheostomy	
D-5 Place an oropharyngeal airway	
D-6 Administer broad spectrum antibiotics pending results of culture and sensitivity	
D-7 Lung expansion therapy (IPPB with normal saline Q4 hours)	
D-8 Bronchodilator therapy (isoetherine Q2 hours)	
D-9 **When you have completed your selections in this section, then develop D-9**	

SECTION E

What would you do now?

Choose only one, unless you are directed to "make another selection in this section".

E-1 Recommend tracheotomy

E-2 Retract the endotracheal tube 3-4 cm

E-3 Increase FIO_2 to 1.0

E-4 Increase FIO_2 to 0.4

E-5 Recommend insertion of chest tube, left hemithorax

SECTION F

The pediatrician requests you make preparations for an intubation attempt. Which of the following would you deem necessary to be present on the intubation tray as you check it, or to have available?

Choose as many as you feel are indicated in this section.

F-1 Endotracheal tube stylette

F-2 Size 2.5 mm ID through 5.0 mm ID endotracheal tubes

F-3 Size 6.0 mm ID through 9.0 mm ID endotracheal tubes

F-4 Succinylcholine for injection

F-5 Laryngoscope, curved and straight tipped blades, battery operative

F-6 Cocaine or xylocaine spray

F-7 Sphygmomanometer

F-8 Valium for injection

F-9 Resuscitation bag connected to 100% oxygen source

F-10 Tube of lubricating jelly

F-11 Suctioning equipment, Yankauer tip catheter

F-12 Large volume, heated nebulizer with 22 mm tubing and T piece (Briggs adaptor)

F-13 A Photospectrometer

F-14 **When you have completed your selections in this section, then develop F-14**

SECTION G

James' drooling has increased, markedly. A stat arterial blood gas is pH 7.34, PCO_2 47 mmHg, PO_2 65 mmHg. Severity of dyspnea has increased. The pediatrician requests you attempt the intubation as she is inexperienced in this procedure. What would you do now?

Choose only one, unless you are directed to "make another selection in this section".

G-1 Attempt the intubation

G-2 Refuse to intubate under any circumstances

G-3 Page the on-call anesthesiologist. He will intubate

G-4 Assure the physician you will make the attempt if she fails.

G-5 Ask the emergency room nurse to intubate

SECTION H

The on-call anesthesiologist arrives several minutes later. After complying with his requests, (ET tube stiffened by insertion of stylette and submerging in ice water). The tube is passed on the first attempt.

What would you include in your post-intubation assessment/treatment of the patient?

Choose as many as you feel are indicated in this section.

H-1 Sputum for acid fast baccilli

H-2 Chest x-ray

H-3 Response to pain

H-4 Institute heated, aerosol therapy via T piece FIO_2 0.28

H-5 Peak inspiratory pressure

H-6 Endotracheal suction

H-7 Chest auscultation

H-8 Postural drainage, percussion, vibration Q4 hours

H-9 Presence of dyspnea

H-10 Chest inspection

H-11 Obtain spirometric data

H-12 **When you have completed your selections in this section, then develop H-12**

SECTION I

Fifteen minutes later James' Dyspnea has increased. Drooling is more evident and he is in panic due to shortness of breath. He is projecting his jaw and keeps pointing to his throat.

Based on this observation, what would be the most likely cause of James' condition?

Choose only one, unless directed to "make another selection in this section".

I-1 Bronchiolitis

I-2 Cystic Fibrosis

I-3 Epiglottitis

I-4 Scarlet fever

I-5 Rubella (German Measles)

SECTION K

During the intubation process, visualization of the glottis is obscured due to swelling, reddening, and edema. Several attempts to pass the tube are unsuccessful.

What would you do now?

Choose only one, unless you are directed to "make another selection in this section".

K-1	Increase FIO_2 to 0.80 Make another attempt	
K-2	Hyperoxygenate with resuscitation bag, FIO_2 1.0. Make another attempt	
K-3	Support ventilation with resuscitation bag, FIO_2 1.0. Call the anesthesiologist for stat intubation.	
K-4	Recommend immediate tracheotomy	
K-5	Insist the attending pediatrician attempt intubation	

James Wilson

Clinical Simulation #9

Answers, Explanations, and Scoring

JAMES WILSON

This pediatric problem tests you knowledge of the physical findings, diagnosis and treatment of epiglottitis. It also places a burden of judgement on your ability to intubate. These intubations are extremely difficult and are best left to an experienced hand—given the gravity of these situations The problem also requires recognition/solution of right mainstem intubation.

SECTION A

Positive Scoring:

A-1 and A-8 Are essential to any assessment.

A-6, A-10, A-11, A-13, and A-14 are key ingredients of a pulmonary assessment.

A-3, A-7, and A-15 are elements of infection. Not only its presence, but also initiating the steps to combat it, if present.

Zero Scoring:

A-4 Although redundant, would neither help nor harm the patient. It would waste time.

Negative Scoring:

A-5, A-9, and a-12 Are procedures not available in an emergency room, nor in a hospital at 9:30 p.m. — unless you did it yourself. The information to be gained would not be of value.

A-2 Urinalysis has no bearing on the immediate respiratory problem.

	Possible	My Score
A-1	+1	
A-2	- 2	
A-3	+1	
A-4	0	
A-5	- 2	
A-6	+2	
A-7	+1	
A-8	+2	
A-9	- 2	
A-10	+1	
A-11	+2	
A-12	- 2	
A-13	+2	
A-14	+2	
A-15	+1	
Total	**15**	

SECTION B

Positive Scoring:

B-4 Is the most logical choice from the information given. The patient is drooling, and his jaw is thrust forward. This is the classic presentation of a child with epiglottitis.

B-3 This choice is forgiveable. The aerosol therapy instituted with oxygen therapy, would relieve dyspnea, somewhat. Croup is usually viral in nature and would not cause an elevated WBC of 13,000 mm^3.

Negative Scoring:

B-1 Is ruled out by normal, vesicular breath sounds. It is also, usually viral in nature, and would not cause stridor—which eminates from the upper airway.

B-2 There is no evidence for this in the patient's history.

B-5 Is ruled out by lack of the usual symptoms leading to pertussis i.e. increased secretions, mucosal edema, sneezing, etc.

	Possible	My Score
B-1	- 3	
B-2	- 3	
B-3	+ 1	
B-4	+ 3	
B-5	- 3	
Total	+ 3	

ALTERNATE ROUTE

SECTION I

Positive Scoring:

I-3 Epiglottitis should be evident. Drooling has increased. There is no response to aerosol therapy and the patient is experiencing increasing severity of upper airway obstruction.

Negative Scoring:

I-1 and I-2 Were explained in the previous section.

I-4 Scarlet fever has a more gradual onset of sore throat, and is also accompanied by rash.

I-5 Rubella also has a more gradual onset of sore throat, fever, and rash.

	Possible	My Score
I-1	- 3	
I-2	- 3	
I-3	+ 1	
I-4	- 3	
I-5	- 3	
Total	**+ 1**	

SECTION C

Positive Scoring:

C-3 and C-4 Documents bacterial infection as opposed to viral infection. The principal infecting organism of epiglottitis is Hemophilus Influenza, a gram (-) bacilli.

C-6 Is a result of a swollen epiglottis and the cause of the drooling.

C-8 and C-9 Definitively identify epiglottitis.

C-10 Depicts alveolar hypoventilation which one would expect with airway obstruction.

Zero Scoring

C-1 A chest x-ray at this point would eliminate the possibility of a foreign body obstruction of the trachea or large airways but is unnecessary in view of the symptoms.

Negative Scoring:

C-2 Would be of no value. It is also hazardous.

C-5 A fluid challenge would require intravenous or central lines. Fluid volume is not in question.

C-7 A lung diffusion study is redundant and not indicated.

	Possible	My Score
C-1	0	
C-2	- 2	
C-3	+ 1	
C-4	+ 2	
C-5	- 2	
C-6	+ 1	
C-7	- 2	
C-8	+ 2	
C-9	+ 1	
C-10	+ 2	
Total	**9**	

SECTION D

Positive Scoring:

Epiglottitis is a medical emergency. The unchecked progression of epiglottic swelling results in complete airway occlusion. Close obervation (D-2) alerting your surgical department for a tracheotomy procedure, (D-4) and commencement of broad spectrum antibiotic therapy (D-6) are imperative. The antibiotic therapy is based on the assumption the causative organism of the infection is hemophilus influenza.

Negative Scoring:

D-1 Is not indicated for epiglottitis.

D-2 Is not indicated.

D-5 An oropharyngeal airway would be rejected by a conscious patient.

D-7 Is also, not indicated nor is D-8.

	Possible	My Score
D-1	- 1	
D-2	+ 2	
D-3	- 2	
D-4	+ 2	
D-5	- 2	
D-6	+ 2	
D-7	- 2	
D-8	- 2	
Total	**6**	

SECTION F

Positive Scoring:

Intubation is the preferred procedure to guarantee a patient airway.

All of the items, except a sphygomomonometer and a photospectrometer, are required before, during and after an intubation.

Negative Scoring:

F-7 and F-13 As above.

F-3 Requires that you recognize 6.0-10.0 mm ID are adult size endotracheal tubes and would be inappropriate.

	Possible	My Score
F-1	+ 2	
F-2	+ 2	
F-3	- 2	
F-4	+ 2	
F-5	+ 2	
F-6	+ 1	
F-7	- 2	
F-8	+ 1	
F-9	+ 2	
F-10	+ 1	
F-11	+ 2	
F-12	+ 1	
F-13	- 2	
Total	16	

SECTION G

Positive Scoring:

It is not prudent for a respiratory therapist to attempt intubation. As the swelling progresses, the normal landmarks disappear and passage of a tube is extremely difficult. James' ABG's indicate some reserve.

G-3 Is the preferable response, although G-1 is forgiveable, particularly is you're background eminently qualifies you to accomplish an extremely difficult procedure.

Zero Scoring:

G-2 Would be unethical presuming you were qualified in the intubation process as described in your hospital and departmental procedure manual.

Many respiratory personnel do not participate in the procedure and are clinically untrained in its implementation. In this case, you are not penalized for this choice.

Negative Scoring:

G-4 Puts undue pressure on an already insecure physician.

G-5 There is no information leading us to believe the emergency room nurse is more qualified than the physician or the respiratory person in attendance.

	Possible	My Score
G-1	+ 1	
G-2	0	
G-3	+ 2	
G-4	- 3	
G-5	- 3	
Total	**+ 2**	

ALTERNATE ROUTE
SECTION K

Positive Scoring:

K-3 Is the preferred response. The attempts have failed. An anesthesiologist (who has been alerted), is the next step short of tracheotomy.

Negative Scoring:

K-1 and K-2 Repeated attempts could cause irrepairable harm to the patient.

K-4 A tracheotomy is major surgery. It should not be performed anywhere other than under sterile conditions, by a surgeon, in a surgical suite. A crycothyroidectomy is the alternative in a dire emergency.

K-5 Is a futile gesture.

	Possible	My Score
K-1	- 3	
K-2	- 3	
K-3	+ 1	
K-4	- 3	
K-5	- 3	
Total	+ 1	

SECTION H

Positive Scoring:

H-2 A chest x-ray is standard procedure post intubation to ascertain proper tube tip position.

H-4 Is also standard procedure to guarantee 100% humidity as well as to add water to the mucociliary elevator following a period of hypoventilation.

H-8, H-9, and H-10 Are also routine prior to obtaining x-ray results. In this case, obviously, something is amiss.

H-7 A routine assessment post intubation.

Negative Scoring:

H-1 A tubercular infection is not in question, hence redundant.

H-3 Response to pain is not only redundant—it is cruel.

H-5 Lung mechanics are also, not in question. The lungs are normal.

H-6 There is no information or evidence secretions need to be removed.

H-11 Is redundant. The lungs are normal.

	Possible	My Score
H-1	-2	
H-2	+2	
H-3	-2	
H-4	+2	
H-5	-2	
H-6	-1	
H-7	+2	
H-8	+2	
H-9	+2	
H-10	+2	
H-11	-2	
Total	**12**	

SECTION E

Positive Scoring:

The evidence uncovered in Section A points to right mainstem intubation. It is within the scope of respiratory practice to correct this situation.

E-2 Will resolve the immediate problem. Epiglottitis responds to antibiotic therapy in two to four days. Presumably James will make a normal recovery, be extubated expeditiously, and on his way home within that period.

Negative Scoring:

E-1 Is to be avoided when alternatives exist. It is major surgery and entails many risks.

E-3 Would lessen dyspnea, possibly, but would not solve the acid-base problems of hypoventilation, nor would E-4.

E-5 The problem of pneumothorax is not evident. James is not being ventilated with positive pressure. It is the right hemithorax not moving, not the left.

	Possible	My Score
E-1	- 3	
E-2	+ 3	
E-3	- 3	
E-4	- 3	
E 5	- 3	
Total	+ 3	

JAMES WILSON

<u>ROUTE</u> <u>SCORING</u>

Route	Possible	My Score
A	15	
B	3	
I	1	
C	9	
D	6	
F	16	
G	2	
K	1	
H	12	
E	3	
TOTAL	**66**	

Optimal Route Passing Score <u>**42**</u>
Alternate Route <u>**43**</u>

REFERENCES

1. Burton, Hodgkins: **Respiratory Care a Guide to Clinical Practice, 2nd Edition,** Lippincott, 1984. (Pages 775-777)

2. Doershuk, Lough, Stern: **Pediatric Repiratory Therapy, 3rd Edition,** Year Book Medical Publishers, Inc., 1985. (Pages 84-85)

Brad Johnson

Clinical Simulation #10

Problem

BRAD JOHNSON
SCENARIO

You are the p.m. shift lead therapist in a 450-bed area medical center. The emergency room charge nurse pages you to assist in the pulmonary care of newly arrived patient. He is a city fireman brought directly to the hospital by his fellow firefighters. They had noticed he was becoming stuperous and incoherent in the course of extinquishing an industrial fire. He is 36 years old. He had just passed his annual physical exam. It is Wednesday, May 15, 1989.

Now go to Section A

SECTION A

Choose as many as you feel are indicated in this section.

On arrival at the emergency room, which would you choose to evaluate?

A-1 Tidal volume, rate and pattern

A-2 Presence of chest pain

A-3 Mental status

A-4 Contents and use of the building—scene of the fire

A-5 Urine output

A-6 Chest auscultation

A-7 Onset of present symptoms

A-8 Inspection of nasal and oropharyngeal mucosa

A-9 Pulse, blood pressure

A-10 Diagnostic chest percussion

A-11 Presence of pedal edema

A-12 Pupillary reflexes

A-13 Chest incursion/excursion

A-14 Odor of breath

A-15 MVV (Maximum voluntary ventilation)

A-16 Clubbing of digits

A-17 Negative inspiratory force

A-18 Jugular vein distention

A-19 Response to painful stimuli

A-20 **When you have completed your selections in this section, then develop A-20**

SECTION B

One hour later, Brad's headache and blurred vision persist, although, he is able to speak lucidly, and walk normally. He requests release so he can return to work. The emergency room physician requests you evaluate the patient's mentation status and cognitive function (ability to think).

What question(s) would be most appropriate to ask?

Choose only one, unless you are directed to "make another selection in this section."

Response

B-1 What year is it?

B-2 Who is our representative to Congress?

B-3 What is the date today?

B-4 What is the sum of 7 + 7?
What is the sum of 14 + 7?
What is the sum of 21 + 7?

B-5 What is the square root of 144?

SECTION C

Thirty minutes later, Brad's level of consciousness has improved. He is now able to sit upright and answer questions. His chief complaint is a severe headache and blurred vision. Which of the following questions would be appropriate to ask to determine the patient's orientation to time and place?

Choose only one, unless you are directed to "make another selection in this section."

Response

C-1 What is your occupation?
Whom do you work for?

C-2 Where are you at?
Who is president of the United States?

C-3 What is your wife's name?
How many children do you have?

C-4 How long have you been married?
Where do you live?

C-5 How old are you?
How old is your father?

SECTION D

The pharmacist determines that forms of cyanide chemicals are used in the electroplating process. He administers amyl nitrate, immediately and leaves a Lily kit for prophylactic treatment for possible cyanide poisoning. It is promptly administered. The patient remains stuperous and is unable to answer your questions. The physician asks if there is any other therapy that would be of benefit to the patient.

What would you recommend now?

Choose only one, unless you are directed to "make another selection in this section."

D-1 Administer aerosol therapy via heated nebulizer

D-2 Hyperinflation therapy (IPPB) 2.5 mg albuterol c 3cc normal saline

D-3 Bronchodilator therapy via hand-held nebulizer

D-4 Administer sodium bicarbonate, continue present therapy

D-5 Intubate and mechanically ventilate

SECTION E

Prior to being called away by another emergency, the physician asks your recommendations for more definitive evaluation of the firefighter's condition.

Which would you perform, evaluate?

Choose as many as you feel are indicated in this section.

E-1 Arterial blood gases

E-2 Sputum for cytology

E-3 Spirometry pre and post bronchodilator

E-4 Serum electrolytes

E-5 CBC

E-6 Carboxyhemoglobin level

E-7 Pharmacologist consult for toxicology profile

E-8 12 lead ECG

E-9 FEV_1/FVC %

E-10 Sputum for inspection

E-11 Chest x-ray

E-12 **When you have completed your selections in this section, then develop E-12**

SECTION F

Which of the following would you monitor while awaiting results of therapy?

Choose as many as you feel are indicated in this section.

F-1 Forced vital capacity

F-2 P50

F-3 Carboxyhemoglobin level

F-4 Orientation to time and place

F-5 Respiratory rate and pattern

F-6 Range of motion

F-7 Level of consciousness

F-8 Arterial blood gases

F-9 General appearance

F-10 Diagnostic chest percussion

F-11 Breath sounds

F-12 Sputum production

F-13 Tidal volume

F-14 Blood pressure

F-15 ECG monitor

F-16 Level of dyspnea

F-17 **When you have completed your selections in this section, then develop F-17**

SECTION G

The emergency room physician arrives. She asks you for a briefing on the situation surrounding the patient's admission, and your best judgement as to the cause of Brad's stuperous condition.

What would be your response?

Choose only one, unless you are directed to "make another selection in this section."

G-1 Myocardial Infarction

G-2 Acute carbon monoxide poisoning

G-3 Pulmonary burns

G-4 Acute carbon monoxide poisoning. There is a possibility of concurrent cyanide poisoning

G-5 Alcohol intoxication

SECTION H

Prior of the arrival of the emergency room physician, who is occupied with another patient, what would be your first course of action?

Choose only one, unless you are directed to "make another selection in this section."

H-1 Administer oxygen via partial rebreather mask

H-2 Administer oxygen via non-rebreather mask

H-3 Administer oxygen 40% venturi mask

H-4 Institute oxygen therapy Nasal cannula, 2 lpm

H-5 Institute aerosol therapy via ultrasonic nebulizer

SECTION I

The emergency room physician returns to see the patient. After a briefing, she asks for your recommendations.

Which would you suggest?

Choose only one, unless you are directed to "make another selection in this section."

I-1 Admit to an intermediate care unit. Continue present therapy.

I-2 Intubate and mechanically ventilate

I-3 Release from the emergency room with okay to return to work

I-4 Admit to the medical intensive care unit institute mask CPAP— 10 cm H_2O FIO_2 0.40

I-5 Refer to the hospital's hyperbaric oxygen service for additional therapy

SECTION J

The hospital hyperbaric oxygen service administered three 90 minute treatments of 100% oxygen at a pressure of 2.5 ATA (atmospheres absolute). At the conclusion of this regimen he requests he be allowed to go home.

Which would you evaluate prior to recommending hospital discharge?

Choose as many as you feel are indicated in this section.

J-1 Serum electrolytes

J-2 Diagnostic chest percussion

J-3 Deep tendon reflexes

J-4 Presence of headache

J-5 Oxygen consumption

J-6 Peak expiratory flow

J-7 Pulmonary capillary wedge pressure

J-8 Level of dyspnea

J-9 Functional residual capacity

J-10 Arterial blood gases

J-11 % Carboxyhemoglobin level

J-12 Response to simple psychometric tests (Serial 7's, Serial 3's)

J-13 Ability to solve simple arithmetic problems (3 x 5, 6 x 3, 4 x 5, etc.)

J-14 **When you have completed your selections in this section, then develop J-14**

SECTION K

Two hours later, Brad still complains of headache and blurred vision. He is also experiencing intermittent nausea with some vomiting. Difficulty with simple psychometric testing persists.

What would you recommend now?

Choose only one, unless you are directed to "make another selection in this section."

K-1 Extracorporeal membrane oxygenation

K-2 Intubate and mechanically

K-3 Commence intercranial pressure monitoring

K-4 Refer to the hospital's hyperbaric oxygen service for further therapy

K-5 Transfer to the hospital's neurologic service for additional therapy

Brad Johnson

Clinical Simulation #10

Answers,
Explanations,
and Scoring

BRAD JOHNSON

This problem requires your management of a carbon monoxide poisoning victim from arrival to discharge. You must treat, diagnose, and be knowledgeable of the long term consequences.

SECTION A

Positive Scoring:

A-1, A-6, A-9, A-10, and A-13 Are all components of a routine respiratory assessment.

A-2, chest pain, and A-14 Are "rule-out" procedures. The patient's presentation could be caused by a heart attack or occult alcohol abuse, or other unusual situations.

It is logical, given the circumstances surrounding the admission (A-7) to think carbon monoxide poisoning, smoke and thermal inhalation (A-8), and gaseous chemical inhalation (A-4).

A-12 The anemic and histotoxic hypoxia is severe.

A-3 Is vital to the assessment as it is indicative of both hypoxia and carbon monoxide inhalation.

Negative Scoring:

A-5 Not only unavailable, but not within the scope of the evaluation.

A-15 Is effort dependent and requires coordination.

A-17 The same as A-15. It, also, is not within the scope of the evaluation. It's, primarily, a weaning procedure.

A-11, A-16, and A-18 Are indicators of COPD and not relevant to the immediate evaluation.

A-19 Under any circumstances, should not be inflicted on a conscious patient.

	Possible	My Score
A-1	+ 1	
A-2	+ 1	
A-3	+ 2	
A-4	+ 1	
A-5	- 2	
A-6	+ 1	
A-7	+ 1	
A-8	+ 1	
A-9	+ 1	
A-10	+ 1	
A-11	- 1	
A-12	+ 1	
A-13	+ 1	
A-14	+ 1	
A-15	- 2	
A-16	- 1	
A-17	- 1	
A-18	- 1	
A-19	- 1	
Total	**13**	

SECTION H

Positive Scoring:

H-2 The optimum response hinges on your knowledge of the FIO_2 delivered by partial rebreather (60-90%), non-rebreather (100%) and a nasal cannula (28%). From your assessment it is safe to assume hypoxia, probably due to carbon monoxide poisoning. The accepted treatment is to administer 100% oxygen immediately.

Negative Scoring:

H-1, H-3, and H-4 Penalize you for your failure to recognize the most probable cause of the fireman's clinical presentation. Adminstering lesser FIO_2's is forgiveable to a lesser degree as you were on the right course.

H-5 Does not address the central problem of hypoxia and would result in great harm to the patient.

	Possible	My Score
H-1	- 1	
H-2	+3	
H-3	- 2	
H-4	- 2	
H-5	- 3	
Total	+3	

SECTION G

Positive Scoring:

G-4 Awards 3 points due to your recognition that carbon monoxide poisoning is frequently accompanied by gaseous cyanide poisoning. Cyanide gas is also a byproduct of burning silk, wool, nylon, fumigating agents and some plastics. The symptoms and treatment are identical to carbon monoxide poisoning.

G-2 Awards 2 points as you have ascertained the central problem.

Negative Scoring:

G-1 Is ruled out as there is no information indicating it a cause. (No chest, arm, etc. pain)

G-3 Smoke/heat inhalation would be indicated if there was evidence of nasal, oropharyngeal burn, as well as the presence of debris. This is not the case.

G-5 Breath odor is negative for alcohol or other fumes (ether, shellac, ketones, etc.) which cause stupor and incoherence. It is not unusual for semi-conscious carbon monoxide poisoning victims to be assumed drunk — particularly in automobiles or motorhomes.

	Possible	My Score
G-1	- 3	
G-2	+ 2	
G-3	- 3	
G-4	+ 3	
G-5	- 3	
Total	**+3**	

SECTION E

Positive Scoring:

E-1 Is not definitive of carbon monoxide poisoning itself. (Note the PO_2) They do define the lactic acidosis which accompanies severe hypoxia at the tissue level. Carbon monoxide poisoning is a combination of anemic and histotoxic hypoxia. It inactivates the cytochrome 3a election chain essential to metabolism of oxygen at the cellular level, as well as, preferentially bind to hemoglobin.

E-6 Denotes the presence of and severity of the poisoning. It is measured by photospectrometer and positively confirms your diagnosis. Some later model ABG analyzers have this capability.

E-7 Is a prudent decision to verify, if present, and determine treatment of, gaseous cyanide inhalation.

E-8 Carbon monoxide poisoning is accompanied by depressed S-Tsegments and erratic P-R intervals.

E-9 and E-11 Verify the absence of smoke or thermal insult.

Zero Scoring:

E-4 and E-5 Could possibly reveal some ancillary problem, but in view of the clinical presentation, would be redundant.

Negative Scoring:

E-2 Cancer is not in question.

E-3 and E-9 Are tests immediately unavailable and the patient unable to perform.

	Possible	My Score
E-1	+1	
E-2	- 2	
E-3	- 1	
E-4	0	
E-5	0	
E-6	+3	
E-7	+2	
E-8	+1	
E-9	- 2	
E-10	+1	
E-11	+1	
Total	**9**	

SECTION D

Positive Scoring:

D-4 The determination of severe metabolic (lactic) acidosis, as noted in Section E, mandates administration of sodium bicarbonate.

Negative Scoring:

D-1, D-2, D-3, as well as D-5 Would not address the problem of metabolic acidosis. The central problem is partially addressed — as you will see as this problem progresses by 100% oxygen at ambient pressures.

Note: A Lily Kit is a prepackaged kit whose principle ingredient is sodium nitrite and sodium thiosulfate when administered intravenously, converts cyanomethemoglobin to thiocyanate — a relatively harmless substance.

Amyl nitrate is administered via the inhalant route to speed the treatment.

	Possible	My Score
D-1	- 3	
D-2	- 3	
D-3	- 3	
D-4	+ 3	
D-5	- 3	
Total	**+3**	

SECTION F

Positive Scoring:

F-3 Denotes progress on the elimination of carbon monoxide from the circulatory system. A maddening facet of carbon monoxide poisoning is that the carboxyhemoglobin level does not always correlate with the clinical presentation of the patient. However, it is central to monitoring the patient.

F-4 and F-7 Are factors to monitor for assessment of the oxygen therapy underway.

F-5 The patient's dyspnea is due to metabolic acidosis. carbon monoxide victims do not, usually, elicit the classic signs and symptoms of hypoxia.

F-8 Is essential to monitor the effects of bicarbonate administration.

F-9 Is essential for monitoring the effects of therapy.

F-15 Is prudent with any patient.

F-16 Is also a progress marker.

Zero Scoring:

F-14 Presumably the patient is monitored and only requires a glance to assess.

Negative Scoring:

F-1, F-10, F-11, and F-13 Are all ventilatory factors which really don't figure into the treatment, assessment, or progress of the patient.

F-2 and F-6 Are not factors for treatment of this patient.

F-12 Sputum is not a factor.

	Possible	My Score
F-1	- 1	
F-2	- 2	
F-3	+ 2	
F-4	+ 1	
F-5	+ 1	
F-6	- 2	
F-7	+ 1	
F-8	+ 1	
F-9	+ 1	
F-10	- 1	
F-11	- 1	
F-12	- 1	
F-13	- 1	
F-14	0	
F-15	+ 1	
F-16	+ 1	
Total	**9**	

SECTION C

Positive Scoring:

C-2 Asks questions which meet the criteria for time and place. Inability to answer, or inappropriate responses are indicators of severe neurological deficit.

Negative Scoring:

C-1, C-3, C-4 and C-5 Are questions that can be answered by conditioned response, despite neurologic deficit.

	Possible	My Score
C-1	- 3	
C-2	+ 3	
C-3	- 3	
C-4	- 3	
C-5	- 3	
Total	**+ 3**	

SECTION B

Positive Scoring:

B-4 This is known as a "serial seven" psychometric test. It goes beyond simple orientation to time and place by requiring the patient to solve simple arithmetic problems. It requires some abstract thought as well as memory.

Carbon monoxide victims, frequently, appear to recover normally, but may be left with serious, long term residuals of the event. They include:

- Recurring headaches
- Vomiting, nausea
- Impaired judgement
- Personality changes

Negative Scoring:

B-1 and B-3 Are answered by conditioned responses.

B-2 and B-5 Are questions most normal people cannot answer.

	Possible	My Score
B-1	- 3	
B-2	- 3	
B-3	- 3	
B-4	+ 3	
B-5	- 3	
Total	+ 3	

SECTION I

Positive Scoring:

I-5 Hyperbaric oxygen therapy is indicated due to the fact Brad is experiencing the conditions which may or may not disappear over a period of time.

To not institute hyperbaric oxygen therapy where it is available would expose Brad to this risk and also expose the hospital to future litigation.

I-1 Is forgiveable, although it would only delay the indicated HBO therapy.

Negative Scoring:

I-2 There are no indications present for intubation and ventilation.

I-3 The problems arising from the event are only partially resolved.

I-4 CPAP is not indicated.

	Possible	My Score
I-1	+ 1	
I-2	- 3	
I-3	- 3	
I-4	- 3	
I-5	+ 3	
Total	+ 3	

ALTERNATE ROUTE
SECTION K

Positive Scoring:

K-4 The time interval, since admission, of 100% oxygen administration is ample to eliminate the presence of carboxyhemoglobin from Brad's hemoglobin. The persistent problems indicate a more ominus situation. Hyperbaric oxygen therapy is the only course open to treat the patient.

Negative Scoring:

K-1 Oxygenation is not the problem.

K-2 There are no indications present for this course of action.

K-3 Is of no value. There is no evidence of increased intracranial pressure.

K-5 There is no treatment (neurologic, or otherwise) to counter the residual effects of carbon monoxide poisoning.

	Possible	My Score
K-1	- 3	
K-2	- 3	
K-3	- 3	
K-4	+ 2	
K-5	3	
Total	+ 3	

SECTION J

Positive Scoring:

J-4, J-12 and J-13 Are appropriate to assess Brad's complete recovery from the poisoning.

J-10 and J-11 Would document a return to normal for hemoglobin, and the lack of metabolic acidosis.

Zero Scoring:

J-8 Would be harmless, but would be, essentially, of little value as it never has been in question since therapy was instituted.

Negative Scoring:

J-1 Has never been in question.

J-2 Is redundant.

J-3 Inflicting pain would be of no help.

J-5 and J-7 Are inappropriate and unavailable.

J-6 and J-9 Are redundant as lung function never has been in question.

	Possible	My Score
J-1	- 2	
J-2	- 1	
J-3	- 2	
J-4	+ 2	
J-5	- 2	
J-6	- 2	
J-7	- 2	
J-8	0	
J-9	- 2	
J-10	+ 1	
J-11	+ 2	
J-12	+ 2	
J-13	+ 2	
Total	**9**	

BRAD JOHNSON

Route	Scoring	
	Possible	My Score
A	13	
H	3	
G	3	
E	9	
D	3	
F	9	
C	3	
B	3	
I	3	
K	2	
J	9	
Total	**58**	

Optimal Route Passing Score **40**
Alternate Route I, K, J Score **41**

REFERENCES

1. Burton, Hodgkins: **Respiratory Care a Guide to Clinical Practice, 2nd Edition,** Lippincott, 1984. (Pages 262-263, 413-414, 889-890)

2. Shapiro: **Clinical Application of Respiratory Care, 3rd Edition,** Year Book Medical Publishers, 1985. (Pages 535-538.

Baby Wells

Clinical Simulation #11

Problem

BABY WELLS

You are a p.m. shift therapist assigned to your hospital's level III neonatal nursery. While doing your first round of ventilator checks, the neonatal charge nurse informs you of a new arrival. It is an approximately 29 week gestational age, 875 gram baby girl. The nurse requests a respiratory evaluation pending the arrival of the neonatologist. The infant was suctioned in the delivery room and has a head hood in place with oxygen to it at 10 lpm.

GO TO SECTION A

SECTION A

Which would you include in your evaluation?

Choose as many as you feel are indicated in this section.

A-1 Temperature

A-2 Pupillary response

A-3 Respiratory rate

A-4 ECG and blood pressure monitor

A-5 Bowel sounds

A-6 Urine color, odor

A-7 12 Lead ECG

A-8 Depth of breathing

A-9 Meconium stain

A-10 Neurologic reflexes

A-11 Sternal retractions

A-12 Tracheal inspection

A-13 Arterial blood gases

A-14 Nasal flaring

A-15 Presence of "grunting"

A-16 Negative inspiratory force

A-17 Chest auscultation

A-18 General appearance

A-19 **When you have completed your selections in this section, then develop A-19**

SECTION B

Appropriate corticosteroid, antibiotic and fluid therapy is ordered and underway. Baby Wells is unstable with episodes of cyanosis, and mottled skin. Tachypnea continues. Which of the following procedures/ modalities would you recommend for the ongoing care of the infant?

Choose as many as you feel are indicated in this section.

B-1 Graphing of compliance measurement Q2 hours

B-2 Placement of an umbilical catheter

B-3 Continuous sodium bicarbonate infusion

B-4 Maintenance of a neutral temperature

B-5 Suction Q2 hours and PRN

B-6 Continuous pulse oximetry

B-7 Sedation of the infant

B-8 Maintain ventilation pressures over 30 cm H_2O

B-9 Maintain P_aO_2 85-95 mmHg

B-10 Continuous aerosol therapy instilled in inspiratory limb of ventilator circuitry

B-11 Apnea monitor

B-12 Arterial blood gases, PRN.

B-13 FIO_2 sufficient to maintain P_aO_2 of 55-75 mmHg

B-14 Postural drainage and percussion Q2 hours

B-15 **When you have completed your selections in this section, then develop B-15**

SECTION C

Fifteen minutes later, another heel stick blood gas is pH 7.26, PCO_2 66 mmHg, PO_2 46 mmHg. Nasal flaring, grunting and tachypnea are still evident.

What would you recommend now?

Choose only one, unless you are directed to "make another selection in this section."

C-1 Ventilate with pressure/time cycled ventilator, FIO_2 0.60

C-2 Increase CPAP to 10 cm H_2O

C-3 Increase CPAP to 15 cm H_2O

C-4 Administer 3 ml of 5% sodium bicarbonate via inhalant route

C-5 Administer racemic epinephrine 0.25 ml in 2 ml normal saline via inhalant route

SECTION D

Based on the information you have gathered, which would you suggest as the most likely cause of Baby Wells' abnormality?

Choose only one, unless you are directed to "make another selection in this section."

D-1 Cerebral intraventricular hemmorrhage	
D-2 Mikity-Wilson syndrome	
D-3 Diaphragmatic hernia	
D-4 Patent ductus arteriosis	
D-5 Infant respiratory distress syndrome	

SECTION E

A sixteen day stay in the neonatal intensive care unit ends for Baby Wells. During that period she was successful in overcoming pulmonary sepsis, potential barotrauma, and was successfully weaned from the ventilator. The neonatal medical staff has made the decision that her parents and siblings are capable of providing home care needed to sustain Baby Wells until prematurity has ceased.

What would you recommend be included in the training of the parents?

Choose as many as you feel are indicated in this section.

E-1 Hyperinflation therapy

E-2 Therapeutic chest percussion and postural drainage

E-3 Drawing of arterial blood gases

E-4 Range of motion exercises

E-5 Sputum evaluation

E-6 Apnea monitoring

E-7 Suctioning procedure

E-8 Operation of a liquid oxygen system

E-9 Spirometry

E-10 Insertion of chest tubes

E-11 Use of nasal CPAP

E-12 Negative inspiratory force

E-13 Performance of Moro-reflex test

E-14 APGAR scoring

E-15 Equipment cleaning techniques

E-16 Administration of aerosolized medications

E-17 Infant CPR

E-18 Feeding precautions

E-19 **When you have completed your selections in this section, then develop E-19**

SECTION F

Which airway would be appropriate to intubate Baby Wells?

Choose only one, unless you are directed to "make another selection in this section."

F-1 An endotracheal tube
7-9 mm ID

F-2 An endotracheal tube
4.0-6.0 mm ID

F-3 An endotracheal tube
2.5-3.5 mm ID

F-4 A carlens tube
2.5-3.5 mm ID

SECTION G

Twenty four hours later, Baby Wells has failed to improve. To determine pathophysiology, which tests/ data would you evaluate?

Choose as many as you feel are indicated in this section.

G-1 P-50 measured

G-2 Chest X-Ray

G-3 Intracranial pressure

G-4 Echocardiogram

G-5 12 Lead ECG

G-6 Complete blood count

G-7 Radial artery blood gas

G-8 Umbilical artery blood gas

G-9 Colorado curve classification

G-10 Daily weight chart

G-11 Thoracic compliance

G-12 **When you have completed your selections in this section, then develop G-12**

SECTION H

The neonatologist arrives. He asks your suggestions as to ventilator parameters.

Which would you recommend?

Choose only one, unless you are directed to "make another selection in this section."

H-1 Assist/control mode, peak pressure 16 cm H_2O, PEEP 5 cm H_2O, FIO_2 0.40, inspiratory time 0.5 seconds

H-2 IMV mode, rate 20, peak pressure, 16 cm H_2O, PEEP 5 cm H_2O, FIO_2 0.40, inspiratory time 0.7 seconds

H-3 Control mode, rate 20, peak pressure 26 cm H_2O, PEEP 10 cm H_2O, FIO_2 1.0, inspiratory time 0.7 seconds

H-4 Control mode, rate 20, peak pressure 36 cm H_2O, PEEP 15 cm H_2O, FIO_2 1.0 sec., inspiratory time 1.0 seconds

H-5 Control mode, rate 20, peak pressure 12 cm H_2O, PEEP 5 cm H_2O, FIO_2 0.60, utilize inverse I:E ratio 1.5:1

SECTION I

Fifteen minutes later, Baby Wells' respiratory rate is 64/minute. Grunting and retractions have increased. The neonatologist communicates via his cellular car phone he is in transit, but is delayed by traffic.

What would you recommend?

Choose only one, unless you are directed to "make another selection in this section."

I-1	Initiate nasal CPAP, 5 cm H_2O, FIO_2 0.60	"Physician disagrees, make another selection in this section"
I-2	Increase FIO_2 to 0.10 via head hood	"Physician disagrees, make another selection in this section"
I-3	Intubate and ventilate via resuscitation bag, FIO_2 1.0	"Physician agrees, go to Section G"
I-4	Intubate, ventilate with pressure/time cycled ventilator, FIO_2 0.60	"Physician agrees, go to Section F"
I-5	Intubate, initiate CPAP 5 cm H_2O, FIO_2 0.60	"Done, go to Section G"

Baby Wells

Clinical Simulation #11

Answers,
Explanations,
and Scoring

BABY WELLS

This problem requires minimal knowledge of standard NICU procedures for monitoring, care, and ventilating policies. It also is necessary to be familiar with current trends in neonatal home care.

SECTION A

The scenario depicts a nine week premature infant. This precludes potential respiratory distress and a host of other problems.

Positive Scoring:

A-3, A-11, A-12, A-13, A-14 , A-15, A-17, and A-18 Are all essential elements of a neonatal evaluation.

A-1, A-4, and A-9 Are secondary elements which would be of value in assessing the infant's respiratory status.

Zero Scoring:

A-7 Is premature, the infant is newly arrived. It could be of value immediately, but it is not helpful nor harmful.

Negative Scoring:

A-2, A-5, A-6, A-10, and A-16 Do not comprise any elements of a respiratory evaluation.

A-8 Would be futile. Neonates cannot regulate breathing by taking deep breaths. They can increase rate only.

	Possible	My Score
A-1	+ 1	
A-2	- 1	
A-3	+ 2	
A-4	+ 1	
A-5	- 2	
A-6	- 2	
A-7	0	
A-8	- 2	
A-9	+ 1	
A-10	- 2	
A-11	+ 2	
A-12	+ 2	
A-13	+ 2	
A-14	+ 2	
A-15	+ 2	
A-16	- 2	
A-17	+ 2	
A-18	+ 1	
Total	**18**	

SECTION I

Positive Scoring:

I-3 This is only a temporary measure and the patient needs mechanical ventilation with PEEP.

I-4 The blood gas values clearly indicate acute ventilatory failure. Intubation and mechanical ventilation are indicated.

I-5 Are indicated to improve oxygenation. It would not addresss the problem of acid-base balance. Either choice will take you on an alternate route.

Zero Scoring:

I-1 This is often protocol, but with patient intubation is the next logical step.

Negative Scoring:

I-2 Would be futile. The blood gas data indicates a refractory P_aO_2.

	Possible	My Score
I-1	0	
I-2	- 3	
I-3	+ 2	
I-4	+ 3	
I-5	+ 1	
Total	+ 3	

SECTION C

ALTERNATE ROUTE

Positive Scoring:

C-1 Is indicated. The blood gas values indicate no significant improvement in ventilatory failure, although the oxygenation status improved somewhat.

Negative Scoring:

C-2 and C-3 Would do nothing to improve hypoventilation, which is the major problem to be overcome.

C-4 and C-5 Are not indicated as there is no evidence of the need for either a bronchodilator/decongestant or a mucolytic.

	Possible	My Score
C-1	+ 1	
C-2	- 3	
C-3	- 3	
C-4	- 3	
C-5	- 3	
Total	**+ 1**	

SECTION F

Positive Scoring:

F-3 Is the proper size range appropriate for this weight infant.

Negative Scoring:

F-2 Is a size range appropriate for pediatric use.

F-1 Are adult sizes.

F-4 Is a double lumen tube for independent ventilation of either the right or left lung. It is not indicated.

	Possible	My Score
F-1	- 3	
F-2	- 3	
F-3	+ 3	
F-4	- 3	
Total	+ 3	

SECTION H

Positive Scoring:

H-1 and H-2 Are appropriate and scored equally. It is prudent to commence ventilation of the neonate at a low pressure. PEEP is indicated due to the refractory nature of the P_aO_2.

A minimum of 0.5 seconds is mandatory to assure adequacy of ventilation. The higher respiratory rates of neonates is the critical factor. Most neonatal ventilators have an independent control to readily regulate inspiratory time.

The FIO_2 is in the safe dosage range.

Negative Scoring:

H-3 Has an excessively high initial peak pressure setting, an excessive oxygen dosage, and inadequate inspiratory time.

H-4 Has the potential for immediate harm to the patient by excessively high pressures delivered to the pulmonary system in general, and the lung parenchyma in particular.

H-5 Contains an inverse I:E ratio. This is indicated only when more conventional ventilatory modes have failed.

	Possible	My Score
H-1	+ 3	
H-2	+ 3	
H-3	- 3	
H-4	- 3	
H-5	- 3	
Total	**+ 3**	

SECTION B

Positive Scoring:

B-2 Until the umbilical artery disintegrates, it is the preferred source of blood gases — which will be required frequently.

B-4 A neonate requires a neutral temperature environment of approximately 99 F. This is accomplished by keeping them on an infra-red warmed table.

B-5 Will be required.

B-6 Is prudent. It is no substitute for arterial blood gases but is an accurate technology to follow swings in oxygenation status of the infant.

B-12 Acid-base status will be the principal means of correctly setting and changing ventilator parameters.

B-13 A P_aO_2 in this range is about as good as you may expect with this degree of prematurity. It is also prudent to avoid excessive FIO_2 delivery.

B-14 Will be required.

Zero Scoring:

B-11 Is not required.

Negative Scoring:

B-1 Is not possible, given the technology of neonatal ventilators.

B-3 Is not indicated.

B-7 Is contraindicated due to its central respiratory control depression.

B-8 ventilation of the neonate entails a very high rate of pneumothorax. 30 CmH_20 is excessive.

B-9 Relates to B-13 above.
It is an excessive range.

B-10 is contraindicated.

	Possible	My Score
B-1	- 2	
B-2	+ 2	
B-3	- 2	
B-4	+ 2	
B-5	+ 2	
B-6	+ 2	
B-7	- 2	
B-8	- 2	
B-9	- 2	
B-10	- 2	
B-11	0	
B-12	+ 2	
B-13	+ 2	
B-14	+ 2	
Total	**14**	

SECTION G

Positive Scoring:

G-2 Is central to determining the specifics of the infant's pathophysiology.

G-4 Is an easily performed, non-invasive means of determining patent ductus arteriosis.

G-5 Would confirm the more definitive tests which pinpoint a patent ductus arteriosis in conjunction with prematurity.

G-7 and G-8 Also confirm the diagnosis. A significantly higher pre-ductal P_aO_2 compared to post-ductal P_aO_2 is a typical of this abnormality.

G-10 Pulmonary edema and fluid retention secondary to congestive heart failure is also typical of this abnormality.

Zero Scoring:

G-6 Could possibly, but not very likely, have some bearing on the problem.

Negative Scoring:

G-1 A hemoglobin abnormality is assumed in the neonate with a left shifted dissociation curve. Measuring it would be redundant.

G-3 Intercranial pressure is not in question.

G-9 Would be of no value. The prematurity is already established.

G-11 Is unobtainable. It also would be redundant as a stiff lung is a part of prematurity.

	Possible	My Score
G-1	- 2	
G-2	+ 2	
G-3	- 2	
G-4	+ 2	
G-5	+ 1	
G-6	0	
G-7	+ 1	
G-8	+ 1	
G-9	- 2	
G-10	+ 2	
G-11	- 2	
Total	9	

SECTION D

From the information gathered in the previous section, patent ductus arteriosis is the central pathophysiology causing the patient's instability.

	Possible	My Score
D-1	- 3	
D-2	- 3	
D-3	- 3	
D-4	+ 3	
D-5	- 3	
Total	+ 3	

SECTION E

Positive Scoring:

E-2 Prematurity necessitates meticulous tracheal hygiene, of which chest physical therapy is a part. This also applies to E-7 and E-15.

E-4, E-6, E-7 and E-15 Are indicated.

E-5 Is essential to warn of pulmonary infections, to which the infant is susceptible.

E-8 Is indicated as the infant will require supplemental oxygen until her lungs mature.

E-16 Is indicated as the infant will require bronchodilators and mulcolytics as needed.

E-17 Cardiopulmonary arrest is a distinct possibility.

E-18 Is required to guard against aspiration.

Negative Scoring:

E-1 Is contraindicated in light of the premature's propensity to pneumothorax.

E-3, E-9, E-10, and E-11 Are procedures for which the parents are completely unqualified.

E-12 Is redundant and unnecessary.

E-13 Is also redundant and unnecessary.

E-14 Is of value only in the immediate post-partium situation.

	Possible	My Score
E-1	- 2	
E-2	+ 2	
E-3	- 2	
E-4	+ 2	
E-5	+ 2	
E-6	+ 2	
E-7	+ 2	
E-8	+ 2	
E-9	- 2	
E-10	- 2	
E-11	- 2	
E-12	- 2	
E-13	- 3	
E-14	- 2	
E-15	+ 2	
E-16	+ 2	
E-17	+ 2	
E-18	+ 2	
Total	**20**	

BABY WELLS

ROUTE AND SCORING

Route	Possible	My Score
A	18	
I	31	
C	1	
F	3	
H	3	
B	14	
G	9	
D	3	
E	19	
Total	**72**	

Optimal Route Passing Score **49**
Alternate Route Passing Score **49**

BABY WELLS

REFERENCES

1. Aloan: **Respiratory Care of the Newborn, A Clinical Manual,** Lippencott, 1987. (Pages 25-97, 135-162, 207-354)

2. Burton, Hodgkins: **Respiratory Care a Guide to Clinical Practice, 2nd Edition,** Lippincott, 1984. (Pages 705-740)

3. Doershuk, Lough, Stern: **Pediatric Respiratory Therapy, 3rd Edition,** Year Book Medical Publishers, Inc., 1985. (Pages 28-48, 54, 55, 59-60, 65-67)

A Note About California College for Health Sciences (CCHS)....

California College for Health Sciences offers vocational and degreed programs in allied health care fields. The school is well known and respected throughout the U.S. for producing unique programs using convenient home-study methods.

The College provides a more flexible alternative to traditional education, with great success. To date, over 10,000 students have graduated. And, as the lifestyle of the '90's continues to demand effective use of limited time, more and more health care personnel will continue to choose CCHS as the way to upgrade their present educational standards..

All CCHS programs are accredited by the Accrediting Commission of the National Home Study Council. Accredidation ensures the school has been carefully evaluated and found to meet standards agreed upon by qualified educators. Only 70 schools in the United States meet NHSC stringent standards.